The Quick and Easy Vegan Air Fryer Delicacies

A Super-easy Recipe Collection to Balance your Lifestyle

Samantha Attanasio

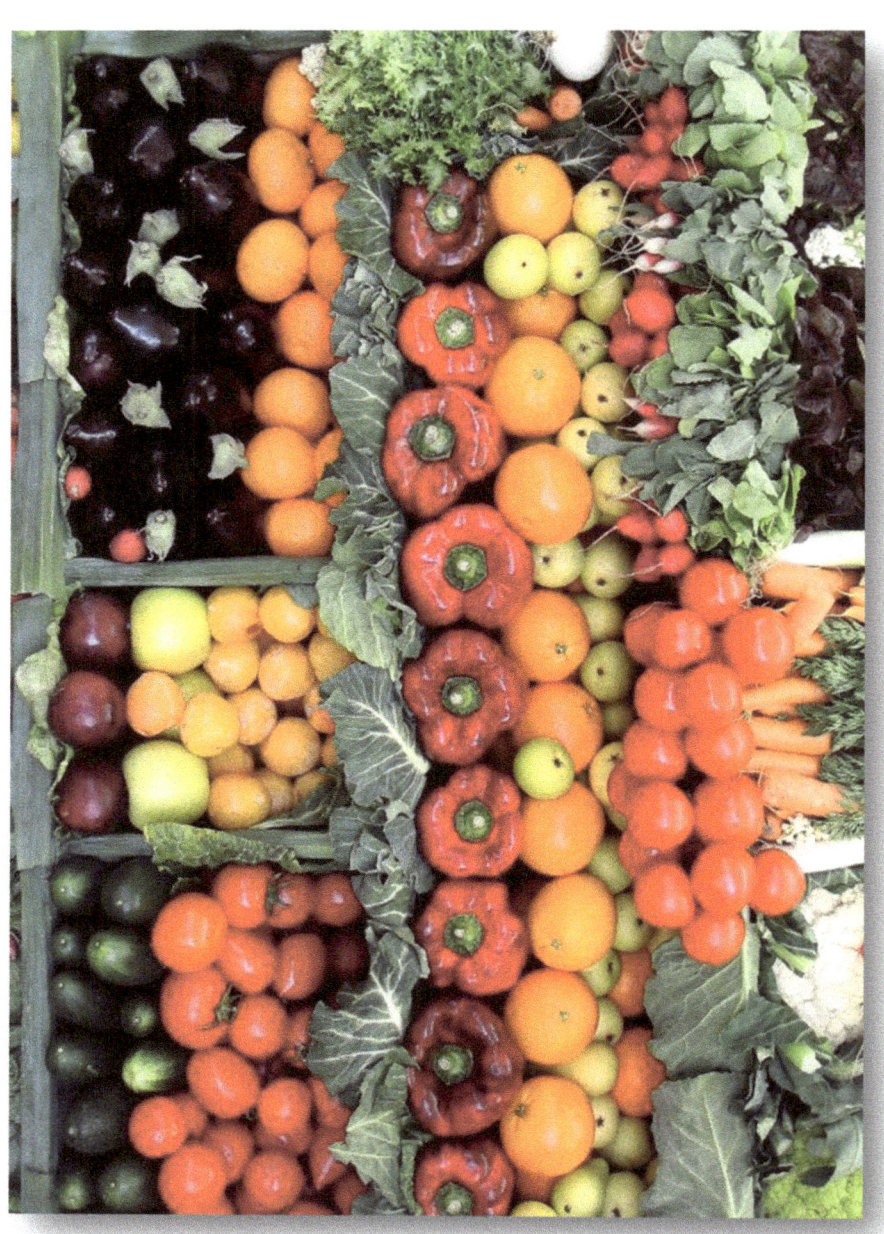

© copyright 2021 – all rights reserved.

the content contained within this book may not be reproduced, duplicated or transmitted without direct written permission from the author or the publisher.

under no circumstances will any blame or legal responsibility be held against the publisher, or author, for any damages, reparation, or monetary loss due to the information contained within this book. either directly or indirectly.

legal notice:

this book is copyright protected. this book is only for personal use. you cannot amend, distribute, sell, use, quote or paraphrase any part, or the content within this book, without the consent of the author or publisher.

disclaimer notice:

please note the information contained within this document is for educational and entertainment purposes only. all effort has been executed to present accurate, up to date, and reliable, complete information. no warranties of any kind are declared or implied. readers acknowledge that the author is not engaging in the rendering of legal, financial, medical or professional advice. the content within this book has been derived from various sources. please consult a licensed professional before attempting any techniques outlined in this book.

by reading this document, the reader agrees that under no circumstances is the author responsible for any losses, direct or indirect, which are incurred as a result of the use of information contained within this document, including, but not limited to, — errors, omissions, or inaccuracies.

Table of Contents

VEGETABLE 7

    Sweet Potato Air Fried Hash Browns 7

    Kale Salad Sushi Rolls 9

    Jackfruit Taquitos 12

    Ginger Tofu Sushi Bowl 14

    Cauliflower Chickpea Tacos 16

    Spicy Cauliflower Stir Fry 18

    Eggplant Parmesan 20

    Stuffed Potatoes 22

    Golden Turmeric Cauliflower Steaks 25

    Golden Turmeric Falafel 27

    Cherry Tomato Salad 29

    Broccoli and Scallions 31

    Balsamic Red Cabbage 32

    Garlic Beans Mix 33

    Oregano Eggplants Mix 34

    Coconut Mix 35

    Artichokes with Coconut 36

    Asparagus and Prosciutto 37

    Cajun Asparagus 39

    Bell Peppers and Kale Leaves 40

    Garlic Parsnips 41

VEGAN FRUITS 42

    Vegan Air Fryer Blueberry Apple Crumble 42

- Vegan Pumpkin Bread Pudding 44
- Cranberry-Carrot Cake 47
- Vegan Gluten-Free Peach Cobbler 49

VEGAN DESSERT 51

- Baked Apples 51
- Blackberry – Apricot Crumble 53
- French Toast with Berries 55
- Peanut Butter – Marshmallow Turnovers 56
- Pigs in a Blanket 58
- Toasted Bread Sandwich 59
- Banana Bread Pudding 60
- Apple Cinnamon Scuffins 63
- Custard and Rhubarb Pie 65

VEGAN SNACKS 67

- Avocado Rolls 67
- Fried Ravioli 69
- Corn Fritters 71
- Mushroom Pizza 73

VEGAN BREAD AND PIZZA 75

- Whole Wheat Vegan Toast 75
- Flat Bread with Olive and Rosemary 78
- Cinnamon Sugar Toast 80
- Salted Caramel Banana Muffins 81
- Pizza Tofu Bites 83

VEGAN MAIN DISHES 85

The Great Taquito 85
The Cheesy Vegan Sandwich 87
Sesame Crunchy Tofu 89

***Vegan Staples* 91**

Korean Fried Tempeh 91
Lemon Tofu Piccata 93
Bbq Lentil Meatballs 96
Cajun French fry Po'boy with Vegan Mushroom Gravy 99
Bbq Soy Curls 102
Buttermilk Battered Tofu 104

Vegetable

Sweet Potato Air Fried Hash Browns

Crispy Air Fryer Hash Browns is a quick, 5-ingredient recipe that is easy, paleo-compatible and Whole-30 compatible. That is a great vegan, low-fat recipe that packs a punch in terms of a flavorful side.

Preparation time: 10 minutes
Cooking time: 20 minutes
Servings: 4

Ingredients:
- Four sweet potatoes, peeled
- Two garlic cloves, minced
- 1 tsp. smoked paprika
- 1 tsp. ground cinnamon
- 2 tsp. olive oil
- Salt and pepper, to tast e

Directions:
Grate the sweet potatoes using the largest side of the cheese box grater.

Place the sweet potatoes in a bowl of cold water and soak for 20-25 minutes. Soaking the sweet potatoes in cold water helps remove starch from the potatoes, which will make them crunchier.

Drain the potatoes and pat dry using kitchen paper.

Place the potatoes in a dry bowl and then add the olive oil, paprika, garlic, salt and pepper. Stir to combine.

Add the potatoes to the air fryer and then cook at 400 degrees Fahrenheit for 10 minutes.

Shake the potatoes at this stage and then cook for a further 10 minutes.

Cool and serve.

Recipe Notes:

Cook times will vary depending on the brand of an air fryer. Check-in on the hash browns after they have cooked for 15 minutes to ensure they do not overcook.

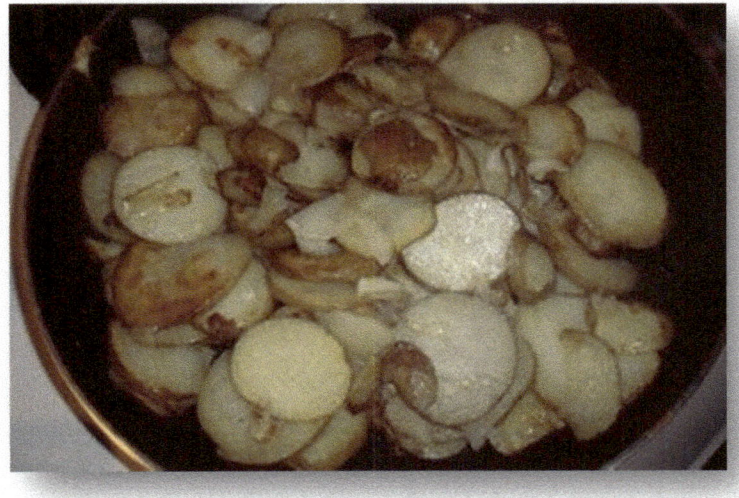

Kale Salad Sushi Rolls

Delicious, crunchy and filling, these Kale Salad Sushi Rolls are easy to make. They're also healthy and flavorful and perfect for entertaining!

Preparation time: 70 minutes
Cooking time: 10 minutes
Servings: 3

Ingredients:
- For the Kale Salad Sushi Rolls:
- One batch Pressure Cooker sushi rice cooled to room temperature
- ½ a Haas avocado, sliced
- Three sheets of sushi nori
- For the Kale Salad:
- 1½ cups chopped kale, de-stemmed
- ¾ tsp. soy sauce
- ¾ tsp. toasted sesame oil
- ½ tsp. rice vinegar
- ¼ tsp. ground ginger
- 1/8 tsp. garlic powder
- 1 tbsp. sesame seeds
- For the Coating:
- ½ cup panko breadcrumbs

- For the Sriracha Mayo:
- ¼ cup of your favourite vegan mayonnaise
- Sriracha sauce to taste

Directions:

To make the Kale Salad:

In a prepared large bowl, combine the kale, sesame oil, vinegar, garlic powder, ginger and soy sauce.

Using clean hands, you can massage the kale until it turns bright green and slightly wilted and then stir in the sesame seeds. Set aside.

To make the Sushi Rolls:

Layout a sheet of nori on a clean and dry surface

With slightly damp fingertips, grab a handful of sushi rice and spread it onto the nori. Try to get a thin layer of rice to cover almost the entire sheet of nori.

Along one edge, leave about ½-inch of naked seaweed; this is the flap that will seal the sushi roll shut.

On the other end of the seaweed, layout 2 - 3 tbsp. of the kale salad, and top with a couple of avocado slices.

Starting with the filling, roll up the sushi roll, pressing gently to get a tight roll.

When in the end, use the naked bit of seaweed to seal the roll shut.

If needed, get your fingertips wet, and then moisten that bit of seaweed to make it stick.

Repeat the steps above to make three more sushi rolls.

To make the Sriracha Mayo:

In a small bowl, whisk together the vegan mayo together with the Sriracha.

Start by adding one tsp. of Sriracha, and keep adding more, half a teaspoon at a time, until the desired spice level is reached.

To fry and slice:

Pour the breadcrumbs into a shallow bowl.

Grab the first sushi roll, and coat it evenly in the Sriracha mayo and then in the breadcrumbs. Repeat for all the sushi rolls.

Place the rolls into the air fryer basket and cook at 390 degrees Fahrenheit for 10 minutes, shaking gently after 5 minutes, to enable them to cook evenly.

When the rolls are cool, take a sharp knife and gently slice them into 6-8 pieces.

When slicing, think of gently sawing and not pressing hard with the knife.

Serve with soy sauce for dipping.

Nutrition:

Energy (calories): 154 kcal

Protein: 2.88 g

Fat: 14.36 g

Carbohydrates: 5.04 g

Jackfruit Taquitos

Air Fryer Jackfruit taquitos are only made of four **Ingredients**, so they are quick and easy to make. What's even better, they only take about half an hour to complete.

Preparation time: 10 minutes
Cooking time: 20 minutes
Servings: 4

Ingredients:
- Four 6-inch corn or whole wheat tortillas
- 1 cup of cooked or canned red kidney beans, drained and rinsed
- 1 14-oz. can water-packed jackfruit, drained and rinsed
- ¼ cup of water
- ½ cup Pico de Gallo sauce
- Canola oil or extra-virgin olive oil cooking oil spray

Directions:
In a medium saucepan, combine the beans, jackfruit, Pico de Gallo and water.
Heat the jackfruit, beans and Pico de Gallo mixture over medium-high heat until it begins to boil.
If you cook on the stovetop, reduce the heat, cover and simmer for 20 - 25 minutes.

If using a pressure cooker, cover it to bring to pressure, cook at low pressure for 3 minutes, and then do a natural release.

Mash the cooked jackfruit with a potato masher to shred the jackfruit to a meaty texture.

Preheat the air fryer at temperature of 370 degrees Fahrenheit for 3 minutes.

Put a tortilla on a clean and dry work surface and spoon a quarter cup of the jackfruit mixture onto the tortilla.

Roll up tightly, putting back any of the mixtures that fall out back into the tortilla.

Repeat this process to make four taquitos in total.

Coat the air fryer basket with the cooking oil spray. Also, spray the tops of the tortillas.

Place the rolled tortillas into the air fryer basket and cook for 8 minutes.

Serve immediately and enjoy!

Nutrition:
Energy (calories): 895 kcal
Protein: 26.8 g
Fat: 26.56 g
Carbohydrates: 140.64 g

Ginger Tofu Sushi Bowl

Ginger Tofu over sushi rice is the perfect low-calorie, a low-fat dish for clean eating. It will fast become your soon-to-be favourite sushi roll fillings.

Preparation time: 10 minutes
Cooking time: 40 minutes
Servings: 4

Ingredients:
- 2-inch piece of fresh ginger
- One clove garlic
- 2 tbsp. real maple syrup
- 1 tbsp. toasted sesame oil
- 2 tbsp. soy sauce
- 1 tsp. rice vinegar
- 1 tbsp. cornstarch (or potato starch)
- One block extra firm tofu pressed and cut into 1-inch pieces
- For the Sushi Bowls:
- One batch Pressure Cooker sushi rice or 3 cups of cooked rice.
- One green onion, sliced
- ¾ cup cucumber sliced into ¼-inch thick half-moons
- ½ cup carrot sticks
- 1 Haas avocado, sliced
- One 0.16-oz packet roast seaweed snacks cut into thirds

- ½ cup roasted cashews
- ¼ cup pickled ginger

Directions:

To make the tofu:

To make the marinade, combine the garlic, ginger, maple syrup, soy sauce, sesame oil, and vinegar in a blender or food processor. Puree on high speed until smooth.

In a large deep bowl, toss together the tofu and the marinade. Set aside and allow to marinate for 10 minutes, then drain any excess marinade.

In the same tub, toss the marinated tofu with the cornstarch. Pour those into the basket of the air fryer and cook at 370 degrees Fahrenheit for 15 minutes. After 8 minutes of Cooking time, shake to make sure they cook evenly.

To make the sushi bowls:

Divide the sushi rice between two bowls.

Top with tofu, green onion, avocado, cucumbers, carrots, seaweed snack pieces and pickled ginger.

Sprinkle on the cashews, and then garnish with the sliced green onion. Serve immediately.

Nutrition:

Energy (calories): 597 kcal

Protein: 21.45 g

Fat: 43.2 g

Carbohydrates: 47.62 g

Cauliflower Chickpea Tacos

Cauliflower Chickpea Tacos are a healthy, fresh and flavorful dinner for all the family. It's quick to get to the table, vegan, easily made and gluten-free.

Preparation time: 10 minutes
Cooking time: 20 minutes
Servings: 4

Ingredients:
- 19-oz. can of chickpeas drained and rinsed
- 4 cups of cauliflower florets, cut into bite-sized pieces
- 2 tbsp. taco seasoning
- 2 tbsp. olive oil
- To Serve:
- Eight small flour tortillas
- 4 cups cabbage, finely shredded
- 2 Haas avocados, sliced
- Coconut yogurt, for drizzling

Directions:
Preheat the air fryer at temperature of 390 degrees Fahrenheit.
In a prepared large bowl, toss the chickpeas and cauliflower with taco seasoning and olive oil.

Put them into the basket of the air fryer and cook in the air fryer for 20 minutes. Make sure to check often to ensure the cauliflower and chickpeas are evenly cooked through.

Serve in tacos with cabbage, avocado slices, and coconut yogurt drizzled on top.

Nutrition:

Energy (calories): 760 kcal

Protein: 22.84 g

Fat: 30.87 g

Carbohydrates: 103.75 g

Spicy Cauliflower Stir Fry

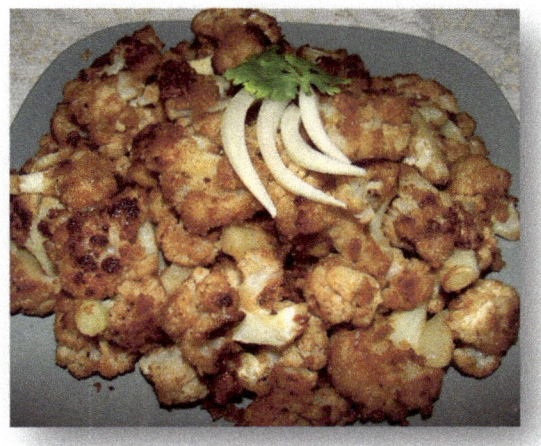

Spicy Cauliflower Stir-Fry is fast, healthy and straightforward. It's so gratifying and works well as a new and exotic side dish for your family to enjoy.

Preparation time: 5 minutes
Cooking time: 25 minutes
Servings: 4

Ingredients:
- One head cauliflower, cut into florets
- Five cloves garlic, finely sliced
- ¾ cup Spanish onion, thinly sliced
- 1½ tbsp. tamari, gluten-free tamari or light soy sauce
- 1 tbsp. Sriracha or any other of your favourite hot sauces
- 1 tbsp. rice vinegar

- ½ tsp. coconut sugar
- To Garnish:
- Two scallions, sliced

Directions:

Place the cauliflower in the air fryer. (If the air fryer has holes in the bottom, you'll need to use an additional air fryer insert).

Preheat the air fryer at temperature of 350 degrees Fahrenheit and cook for 10 minutes.

Open the air fryer, remove and shake the insert and slide back into the compartment.

Add the sliced white onion, stir and cook for a further 10 minutes.

Attach the garlic, then stir and cook for an additional five minutes.

In a small bowl, mix the rice vinegar, soy sauce, coconut sugar, Sriracha hot sauce, salt and pepper.

Add the mixture to the cauliflower in the air fryer and stir—Cook for a further 5 minutes. The insert will keep all of the juices inside.

Transfer to a serving bowl and then sprinkle the sliced scallions over the top to garnish.

Nutrition:

Calories: 93 kcal.

Carbohydrates 12g

Total Fat 3g

Protein 4g

Sodium 510mg

Potassium 519mg

Eggplant Parmesan

This easy Italian vegetarian dish, Eggplant Parmesan, is the perfect light weekday dinner. And made in the air-fryer, it couldn't be easier!

Preparation time: 10 minutes
Cooking time: 20 minutes
Servings: 6

Ingredients:
- One large eggplant, sliced and de-stemmed
- ½ cup almond milk
- ½ cup flour
- 2 tbsp. vegan Parmesan, grated
- ½ cup Panko bread crumbs
- Garlic powder, to taste
- Onion powder, to taste
- Salt and pepper, to taste
- For the Topping:
- 1 cup of Marinara sauce, plus more for serving
- Vegan Parmesan, grated
- ½ cup Vegan Mozzarella Shreds
- To Serve:
- 4 oz. spaghetti or any other pastas your desired, cooked al dente (to serve two people)

- Vegan Parmesan, grated
- Italian parsley, chopped

Directions:

Wash, dry, de-stem the eggplant and slice lengthways.

Season the Panko breadcrumbs with vegan parmesan, garlic powder, onion powder, salt and pepper.

Dip the sliced eggplant into the flour, and then the almond milk and finally, the seasoned Panko bread crumbs.

Spray the eggplant lightly with cooking oil spray and place into the air fryer basket at 390 degrees Fahrenheit for 15 minutes. Check the eggplant flipping halfway through cooking, flip over and spray the second side lightly with cooking oil spray.

Nutrition:

Energy (calories): 146 kcal

Protein: 7.2 g

Fat: 3.13 g

Carbohydrates: 23.71 g

Stuffed Potatoes

Scrumptious and filling! This baked potato filled with a cheesy mash and re-baked will have your family asking for more. The air fryer can make the whole cooking process go faster and crisping up the potato even more. Try it out today!

Preparation time: 10 minutes
Cooking time: 90 minutes
Servings: 4

Ingredients:
- Two large Russet baking potatoes
- 1 - 2 tsp. olive oil (you may leave the oil out if you want the recipe oil-free)
- 1 cup spinach or kale, chopped
- 2 tbsp. Nutritional yeast
- ¼ cup unsweetened almond milk
- ¼ cup unsweetened vegan yogurt
- ½ tsp. salt
- ¼ tsp. pepper
- For Topping (Optional):
- Smoked salt and black pepper, to taste
- Chopped chives, parsley or any other of your favourite fresh herbs
- ¼ cup unsweetened vegan yogurt

Directions:

Rub the skin of each Russet potato with oil on all sides.

Preheat the air fryer at the temperature of 390 degrees Fahrenheit unless the brand doesn't require it.

Once it's hot, add the potatoes to the air fryer basket.

Cook the potatoes for 30 minutes, and when the time is up, flip the potatoes over and cook for 30 more minutes.

Depending on the potatoes' size, they may need to cook for a further 10 - 20 minutes. The potatoes will be fork tender when it is already cooked. Set them aside to cool.

Slice each potato into half lengthwise and then scoop out the flesh while leaving enough to create a stable shell of the potato skin.

Mash the scooped potato flesh, almond milk, vegan yogurt, Nutritional yeast, pepper and salt until smooth.

Then stir in the chopped spinach and fill the potato shells.

Cook the filled potatoes again at 350 degrees Fahrenheit for 5 minutes.

Serve with the toppings you really enjoy!

If you don't have an air fryer to use, you can do this all in the oven at 400 degrees Fahrenheit. Cooking times may vary since the air fryers use a convection type cooking method.

While the eggplant is cooking, for the meantime cook the pasta.

Once golden on both sides, spoon some of the marinara sauce on top of the eggplant and top with a combination of the vegan Parmesan and mozzarella cheeses. Cook just until the cheeses just begin to melt.

Serve with the pasta, extra Marinara. Garnish with fresh parsley and perhaps another sprinkle of the vegan parmesan. Enjoy!

Nutrition:

Energy (calories): 211 kcal

Protein: 7.64 g

Fat: 3.24 g

Carbohydrates: 38.47 g

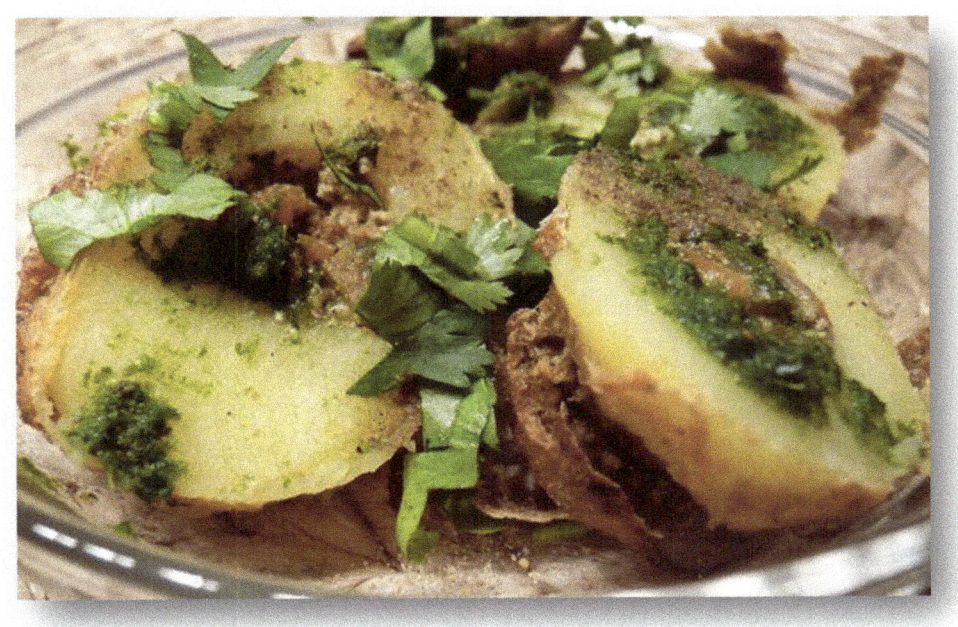

Golden Turmeric Cauliflower Steaks

These healthy, meaty and delicious golden turmeric Cauliflower Steaks are loaded with flavor and full of spice. Perfect for a light lunch or dinner.

Preparation time: 10 minutes
Cooking time: 15 minutes
Servings: 2

Ingredients:
- 1-2 medium heads cauliflower, stems intact
- 2 tbsp. coconut oil or coconut spray Oil
- 1 tsp. ground turmeric
- ¼ tsp. ground ginger
- 1/8 tsp. ground cumin
- 1/8 tsp. salt
- A pinch of black pepper
- To Serve:
- Mixed steamed greens
- Tahini
- White Sesame Seeds

Directions:

Cut the cauliflower head down the middle, leaving the stem intact. Trim off any green leaves.

On either side of the half, cut 1-inch steaks taking care not to make them too thin. Reserve any fallen florets for use at a later date.

Coat the steaks with coconut oil or coconut oil spray and rub the spices into all of the cauliflower cracks and crevices.

These recipes can be prepared in the oven or an air fryer. Cook at 390 degrees Fahrenheit for about 15 minutes, turning over the steaks halfway through the Cooking time.

Serve the mixed greens on a bed, drizzled with tahini. Garnish with white sesame seeds, if desired.

Nutrition:

Energy (calories): 185 kcal

Protein: 4.46 g

Fat: 14.29 g

Carbohydrates: 13.26 g

Golden Turmeric Falafel

Preparation time: 15 minutes
Cooking time: 20 minutes
Servings: 4

Ingredients:
- For the falafel:
- 1 cup canned chickpeas, drained and rinsed
- 2 tbsp. tahini
- 2 tbsp. white onion, diced
- ½ tsp. fresh garlic, minced
- 2 tbsp. lemon juic e
- 2 tbsp. fresh parsley
- 1 tsp. ground turmeric
- ½ tsp. ground cumin
- ¼ tsp. salt
- 1/8 tsp. black pepper
- For the tzatziki dipping sauce:
- ¼ cup cucumber, finely diced
- One container vegan almond milk yogurt
- 2 tsp. lemon juice
- 1 tsp. dill
- Salt & Pepper, to taste
- Garlic powder, to taste
- For the couscous tabbouleh:

- ¼ cup chickpeas that remain from the falafel preparation 1 cup cooked quinoa or couscous
- 2 tbsp. cucumber, diced
- 2 tbsp. tomato, diced
- One green onion, diced
- 2 tbsp. fresh parsley
- Salt & pepper, to taste

Directions:

Preheat the air fryer at temperature of 370 degrees Fahrenheit or, if using an oven, 375 degrees Fahrenheit.

In a food processor, now combine all the falafel Ingredients and carefully pulse until all the Ingredients are coarsely chopped but mixed well.

Coat the air fryer basket with vegan cooking oil spray.

Using an ice cream scoop, scoop four balls of the mixture and flatten them into patties in your hands

Air fry (or bake in the oven) for 15 minutes. Halfway through cooking, flip them over to ensure even cooking.

While the falafel is cooking, prepare the couscous salad and tzatziki using all the Ingredients.

Serve garnished with a few lemon wedges and fresh parsley.

Nutrition:

Energy (calories): 165 kcal

Protein: 7.39 g

Fat: 5.81 g

Carbohydrates: 23.37 g

Cherry Tomato Salad

Preparation time: 5 minutes
Cooking time: 25 minutes
Servings: 6

Ingredients:
- Eight small beets, trimmed, peeled and cut into wedges
- One red onion, sliced
- One tbsp. balsamic vinegar
- Salt and black pepper to taste
- 1 pint mixed cherry tomatoes, halved
- 2 ounces pecans, chopped
- Two tbsp. olive oil

Directions:
Put the beets in your air fryer's basket, and add the salt, pepper, and one tbsp. of the oil.
Cook at the temperature of 400 degrees F for 15 minutes.
Transfer the beets to a pan that fits your air fryer, and add the onions, tomatoes, pecans, and remaining one tbsp. of the oil; toss well.
Cook at 400 degrees F for ten more minutes.
Divide between plates and serve.

Nutrition:
Calories 144
Fat 7g

Fiber 5g
Carbs 8g
Protein 6g

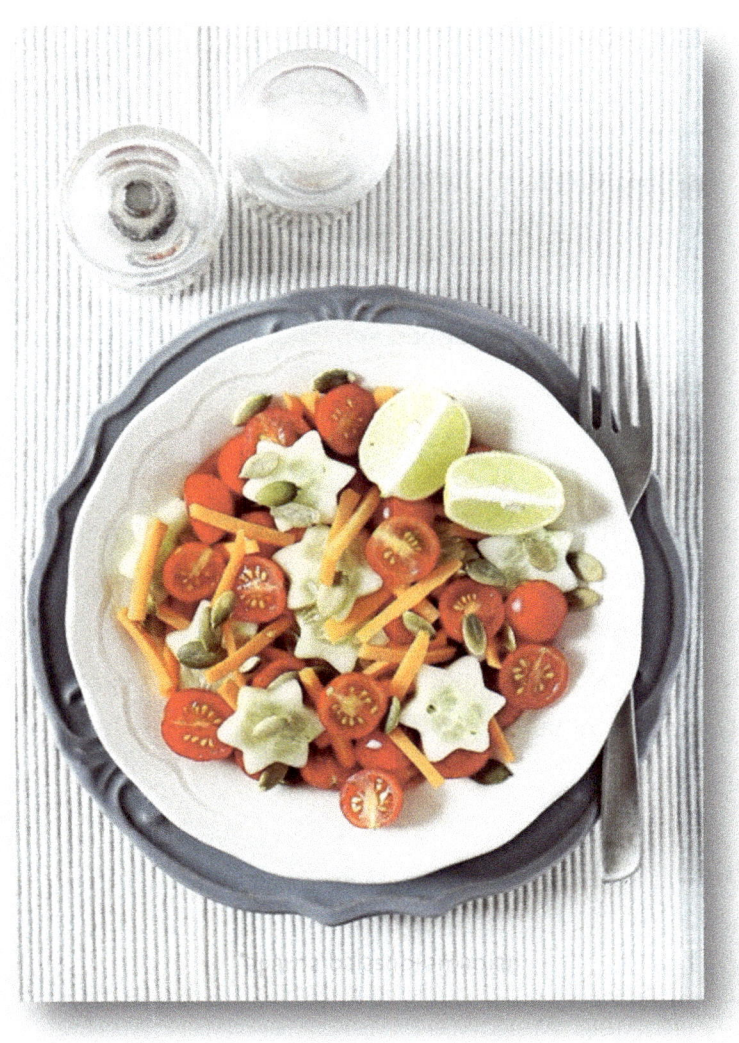

Broccoli and Scallions

Preparation time: 5 minutes
Cooking time: 7 minutes
Servings: 4

Ingredients:
- One broccoli head, florets separated
- Salt and black pepper to taste
- Six cherry tomatoes, halved
- ¼ cup scallions, chopped
- One tbsp. olive oil

Directions:
Put the broccoli florets in your air fryer's basket, and add the salt, pepper, and ½ tbsp. of the oil; toss well.
Cook at 380 degrees F for 7 minutes .
Transfer the broccoli to a bowl, and add the tomatoes, scallions, salt, pepper, and the remaining ½ tbsp. of oil.
Toss and serve.

Nutrition:
Calories 111
Fat 4g
Fiber 4g
Carbs 9g
Protein 2g

Balsamic Red Cabbage

Preparation time: 5 minutes
Cooking time: 8 minutes
Servings: 4

Ingredients:
- One red cabbage head, shredded
- One tbsp. olive oil
- One carrot, grated
- ¼ cup balsamic vinegar
- Salt and black pepper to taste
-

Directions:
Place all Ingredients in a pan that fits your air fryer, and mix well. Put the pan in the fryer and cook at 380 degrees F for 8 minutes. Divide between plates and serve.

Nutrition:
Calories 100
Fat 4g
Fiber 2g
Carbs 7g
Protein 2g

Garlic Beans Mix

Preparation time: 5 minutes
Cooking time: 6 minutes
Servings: 4

Ingredients:
- 1 pound green beans, trimmed
- Two tbsp. olive oil
- Three garlic cloves, minced
- Salt and black pepper to taste
- One tbsp. balsamic vinegar

Directions:
Place all the Ingredients in a prepared bowl, except the vinegar, and mix well.
Put the beans in your air fryer and cook at 400 degrees F for 6 minutes.
Divide the green beans between plates, drizzle the vinegar all over, and serve.

Nutrition:
Calories 101
Fat 3g
Fiber 3g
Carbs 4g
Protein 2g

Oregano Eggplants Mix

Preparation time: 5 minutes
Cooking time: 15 minutes
Servings: 4

Ingredients:
- Four eggplants, roughly cubed
- Two tbsp. lime juice
- Salt and black pepper to taste
- One tsp. oregano, dried
- Two tbsp. olive oil

Directions:

Place all of Ingredients together in a pan that fits your air fryer and mix/toss well.

Put the pan into the fryer and cook at 400 degrees F for 15 minutes.

Divide the eggplants between plates and serve.

Nutrition:

Calories 125

Fat 5g

Fiber 2g

Carbs 11g

Protein 5 g

Coconut Mix

Preparation time: 5 minutes
Cooking time: 8 minutes
Servings: 8

Ingredients:
- 1 pound brown mushrooms, halved
- One small yellow onion, chopped
- Salt and black pepper to taste
- Two tbsp. olive oil
- 14 ounces of coconut milk

Directions:
Add all Ingredients to a pan that fits your air fryer and mix well . Place the pan in the fryer and cook at 400 degrees F for 8 minutes. Divide between plates and serve.

Nutrition:
Calories 202
Fat 4g
Fiber 1g
Carbs 13g
Protein 4g

Artichokes with Coconut

Preparation time: 5 minutes
Cooking time: 15 minutes
Servings: 2

Ingredients:
- Two artichokes, washed, trimmed and halved
- Two garlic cloves, minced
- ¼ cup coconut, shredded
- Juice of 1 lemon
- One tbsp. coconut oil, melted
-

Directions:
In a bowl, mix the artichokes with the garlic, oil, and lemon juice; toss well.
Put the artichokes into your air fryer and cook at 360 degrees F for 15 minutes.
Divide the artichokes between plates, sprinkle the coconut on top, and serve.
Enjoy!

Nutrition:
Calories 213
Fat 8g
Fiber 6g
Carbs 13g
Protein 6g

Asparagus and Prosciutto

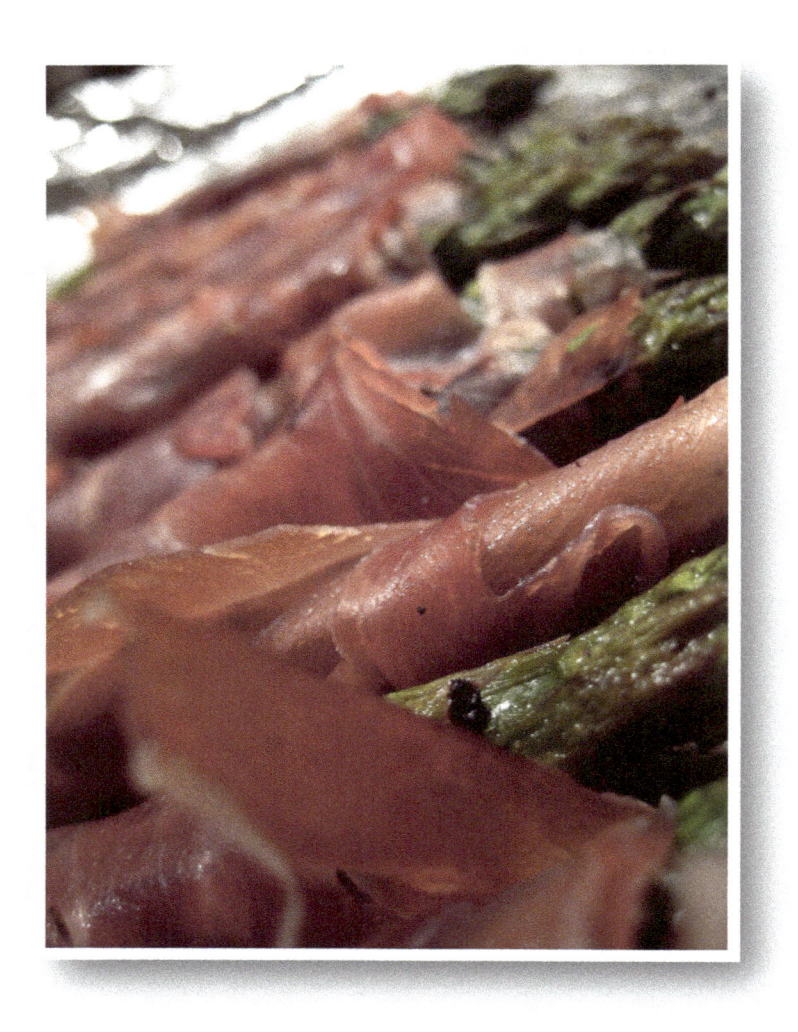

Preparation time: 5 minutes
Cooking time: 5 minutes
Servings: 4

Ingredients:
- Eight asparagus spears, trimmed
- 8 ounces prosciutto slices
- A pinch of salt and black pepper

Directions:

Wrap the asparagus in prosciutto slices and then season with salt and pepper.

Put all in your air fryer's basket and cook at 400 degrees F for 5 minutes.

Divide between plates and serve.

Nutrition:

Calories 100

Fat 2g

Fiber 5g

Carbs 8g

Protein 4g

Cajun Asparagus

Preparation time: 5 minutes
Cooking time: 5 minutes
Servings: 4

Ingredients:
- One tsp. extra virgin olive oil
- One bunch asparagus, trimmed
- ½ tbsp. Cajun seasoning

Directions:
In a prepared bowl, mix the asparagus with the oil and Cajun seasoning; coat the asparagus well.
Put the asparagus in your air fryer and cook at 400 degrees F for 5 minutes.
Divide between plates and serve.

Nutrition:
Calories 151
Fat 3
Fiber 4
Carbs 9
Protein 4

Bell Peppers and Kale Leaves

Preparation time: 5 minutes
Cooking time: 15 minutes
Servings: 4

Ingredients:
- Two red bell peppers, cut into strips
- Two green bell peppers, cut into strips
- ½ pound kale leaves
- Salt and black pepper to taste
- Two yellow onions, roughly chopped
- ¼ cup veggie stock
- Two tbsp. tomato sauce

Directions:
Add all Ingredients to a pan that fits your air fryer; mix well.
Place the pan in the fryer and cook at 360 degrees F for 15 minutes.
Divide between plates, serve, and enjoy!

Nutrition:
Calories 161
Fat 7g
Fiber 6g
Carbs 12g
Protein 7g

Garlic Parsnips

Preparation time: 5 minutes
Cooking time: 15 minutes
Servings: 4

Ingredients:
- 1 pound parsnips, cut into chunks
- One tbsp. olive oil
- Six garlic cloves, minced
- One tbsp. balsamic vinegar
- Salt and black pepper to taste

Directions:
In a prepared bowl, add all of the Ingredients and combine well. Place them in the air fryer and cook at 380 degrees F for 15 minutes. Divide between plates and serve.

Nutrition:
Calories 121
Fat 3g
Fiber 6g
Carbs 12g
Protein 6g

Vegan Fruits

Vegan Air Fryer Blueberry Apple Crumble

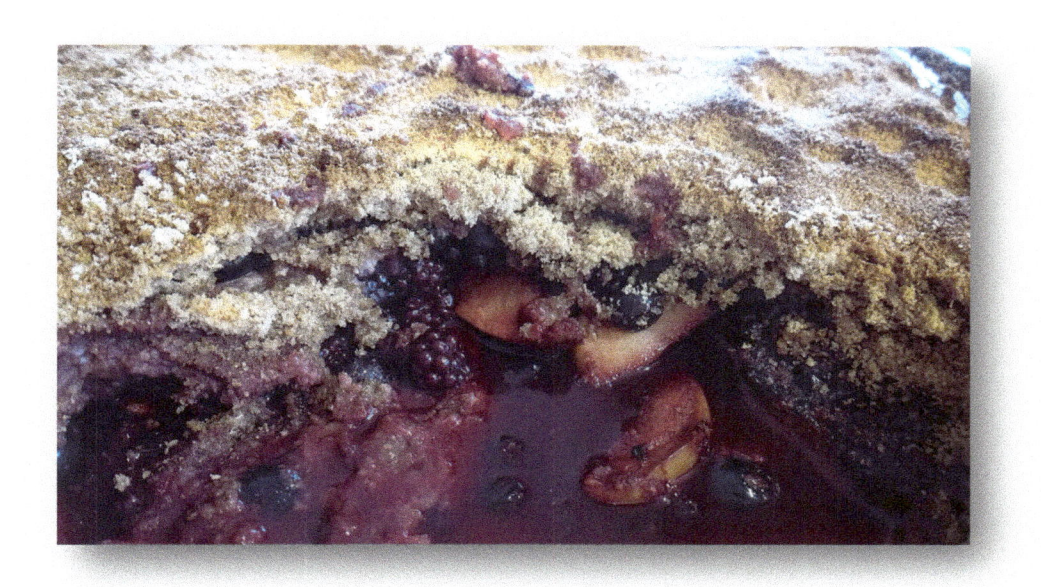

Preparation time: 10 minutes
Cooking time: 20 minutes
Servings: 4

Ingredients:
- 1 medium apple, finely diced
- ½ cup frozen blueberries, strawberries, or peaches

- ¼ cup plus one tbsp. brown rice flour
- 2 tbsp. sugar
- ½ tsp. ground cinnamon
- 2 tbsp. non-dairy butter

Directions:

Preheat the air fryer set 5 minutes to 350 ° F. Mix the apple and frozen blueberries in a healthy baking pan or ramekin air fryer.

In a prepared small bowl, combine the flour, sugar, cinnamon, and butter. Spoon the flour mixture over the fruit. Sprinkle a little extra flour over everything to cover any exposed fruit—Cook at 350°F for 15 minutes.

Nutrition:

Energy (calories): 128 kcal

Protein: 2.18 g

Fat: 4.43 g

Carbohydrates: 21.7 g

Vegan Pumpkin Bread Pudding

Preparation time: 10 minutes
Cooking time: 50 minutes
Servings: 4

Ingredients:
- 1 16 ounces loaf French bread
- ½ cup raisins
- 1 ½ cup of soymilk or other non-dairy milk vanilla or plain
- 1 cup of pumpkin canned or cooked and pureed
- ¼ cup maple syrup
- ¼ cup dark brown sugar
- 1 tbsp. Ener-G Egg Replacer may substitute 2 ½ tsp. Starch (tapioca, potato, or corn starch) plus ½ tsp. baking powder
- 2 tsp. vanilla extract
- 1 ½ tsp. cinnamon
- ½ tsp. ginger powder
- ½ tsp. nutmeg
- ¼ tsp. allspice
- 1/8 tsp. ground cloves
- ¼ tsp. salt optional
- Sauce
- ½ cup apple cider or juice
- ¼ cup maple syrup
- 1 tsp. cornstarch mixed with one tbsp. apple juice

- 1 ½ tbsp. brandy, rum, or bourbon add to taste up to ¼ cup
- ¼ cup chopped pecans or walnuts optional

Directions:

Cut or slice the bread into bite-sized pieces. If the bread looks moist or dense, spread it out on a cookie sheet and toast it for a few minutes in the oven. Place it in a large bowl and add the raisins.

Put the non-dairy milk into the blender along with the pumpkin, maple syrup, sugar, Ener-G, vanilla, spices, and salt. Blend until smooth. Pour it over the bread, using a silicone spatula to get out every drop. Stir well to coat all of the bread thoroughly. Set aside then soak for a few minutes while you ready the pan and preheat the oven.

Preheat oven to 350F. Line an 8x8-inch baking dish with parchment paper or foil lightly. Pour the bread pudding into the pan in an even layer. Bake for about 45 minutes or until the top is set and beginning to brown. Remove from oven and allow cooling for at least 15 minutes. While the pudding is cooling, make the sauce. Place the apple cider and the maple syrup in a small saucepan over medium heat, and bring to a simmer, often stirring, until reduced to about half.

Carefully add the cornstarch mixture, bring it to a boil, and cook for another couple of minutes, continually stirring until the mix is no longer cloudy and thickens slightly. Remove from heat and add the brandy or other spirits a little at a time, to taste. Stir in the nuts. Poke a few holes in the top of the bread pudding with a toothpick, and pour the sauce over the top, distributing nuts evenly. Cut into squares and serve warm.

Nutrition:

Energy (calories): 1579 kcal

Protein: 21.89 g

Fat: 102.42 g

Carbohydrates: 102.05 g

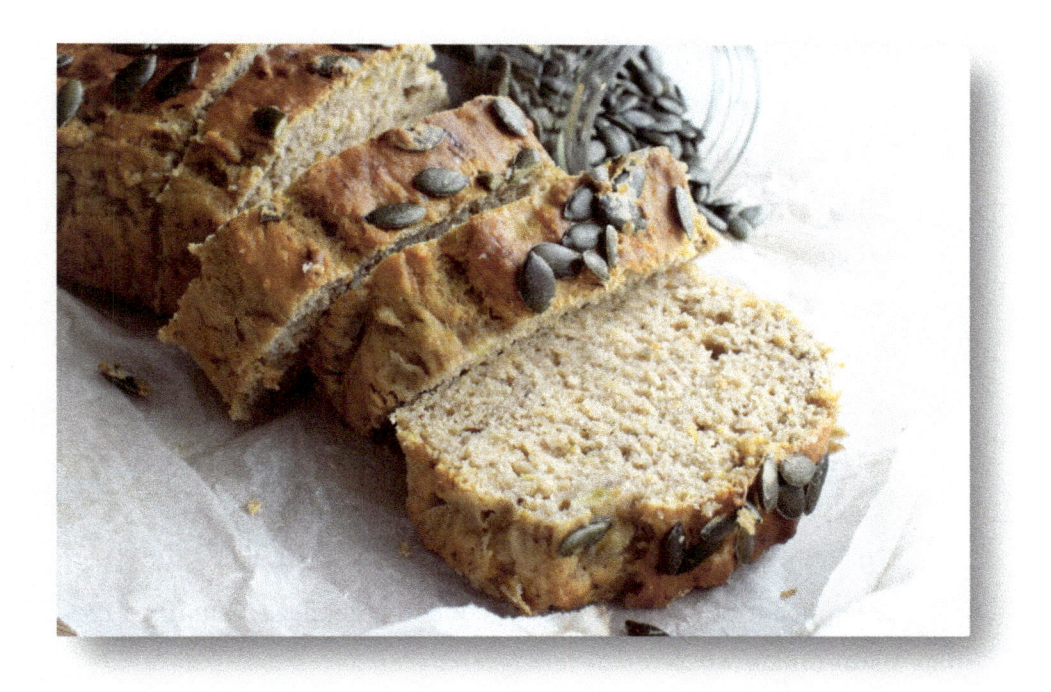

Cranberry-Carrot Cake

Preparation time: 10 minutes
Cooking time: 40 minutes
Servings: 4

Ingredients:

- 8-10 ounces fresh cranberries
- 1/3 cup natural granulated sugar
- 1 ¾ cups whole wheat pastry flour (or white whole wheat flour)
- 2 tbsp. ground flaxseeds
- 1 tsp. baking powder
- ½ tsp. baking soda
- ½ tsp. ground ginger
- ½ tsp. cinnamon
- ½ cup applesauce
- 1/3 cup maple syrup
- 2 tbsp. (liquid from canned or cooked chickpeas) aquafaba or plant milk of choice
- 1 tsp. vanilla extract
- 1 cup of grated carrot
- Maple-Cream Cheese frosting optional (see recipe in Notes)
- 1/3 cup finely chopped walnuts optional
- Confectioner's sugar optional

Directions:

Place the cranberries in a blade-fitted food processor and pulse on and off until chopped evenly and finely. Switch to a tub. Add the sugar, whisk thoroughly, and set aside.

Preheat oven to 350F.

In a large mixing bowl, combine the flour, flaxseeds, baking powder, baking soda, ginger, and cinnamon. Stir to combine thoroughly.

Make a hole in the center then add the applesauce, syrup, aquafaba/plant milk, and vanilla. Stir until the wet and dry Ingredients are thoroughly combined, but don't over mix. Stir the batter with the cranberries and carrots.

Pour into a 9-inch circular cake pan with silicone. Springform pan or lightly oiled pan (see headnote). Bake for 35 to 40 minutes, or until the knife comes out clean inserted in the middle.

If using the walnuts, toast them in a small dry skillet over medium heat until they brown lightly.

If you have used a springform or other easy-to-release pan, release the pan once the cake has cooled to room temperature and spread the frosting evenly over the surface, allowing it to drip over the sides. Otherwise, in the pan, leave the cake and simply frost the top.

(If you don't wish to use the frosting, you can sprinkle the top with confectioners' sugar or just serve it plain.) With the optional walnuts, sprinkle evenly and then cut into wedges to serve.

Nutrition:

Energy (calories): 416 kcal

Protein: 9.37 g

Fat: 8.22 g

Carbohydrates: 81.3 g

Vegan Gluten-Free Peach Cobbler

Preparation time: 10 minutes
Cooking time: 40 minutes
Servings: 4

Ingredients:
- Peaches
- 2 pounds peaches (about five large)
- 1 tsp. lemon juice
- 2 tbsp. sugar
- ¼ tsp. cinnamon optional
- Dry
- 1 cup gluten-free baking flour blend
- ½ cup sugar
- 2 tbsp. tapioca starch (also called tapioca flour)
- 1 tbsp. baking powder
- Pinch salt
- Wet
- ¾ cup soy milk or other non-dairy milk
- ½ tsp. vanilla extract

Directions:

Bring several inches of water and let it boil in a large saucepan. Use a slotted spoon to lower each peach into the boiling water for about 20 seconds. Place on a cutting board or plate and set aside to cool. (This makes the peaches easy to peel.)

When the peaches are cool enough, peel them by piercing the skin with a knife and pulling it off. Slice the peaches into a large bowl. Add the lemon juice, two tbsp. Of sugar and cinnamon, if desired .

Preheat Air fryer set to 375 degrees F. Arrange the peaches in a deep 9-inch pie pan.

Mix the dry Ingredients. Then add the wet Ingredients, and stir just enough to eliminate large lumps. Pour over the peaches.

Bake for 35-45 minutes, covering loosely with aluminum foil if the top begins to get too brown. It's done with you can stick a toothpick in the middle and not have batter attached to it.

Allow cooling for a few minutes before serving.

Nutrition:

Energy (calories): 745 kcal

Protein: 6.81 g

Fat: 58.71 g

Carbohydrates: 51.99 g

Vegan Dessert

Baked Apples

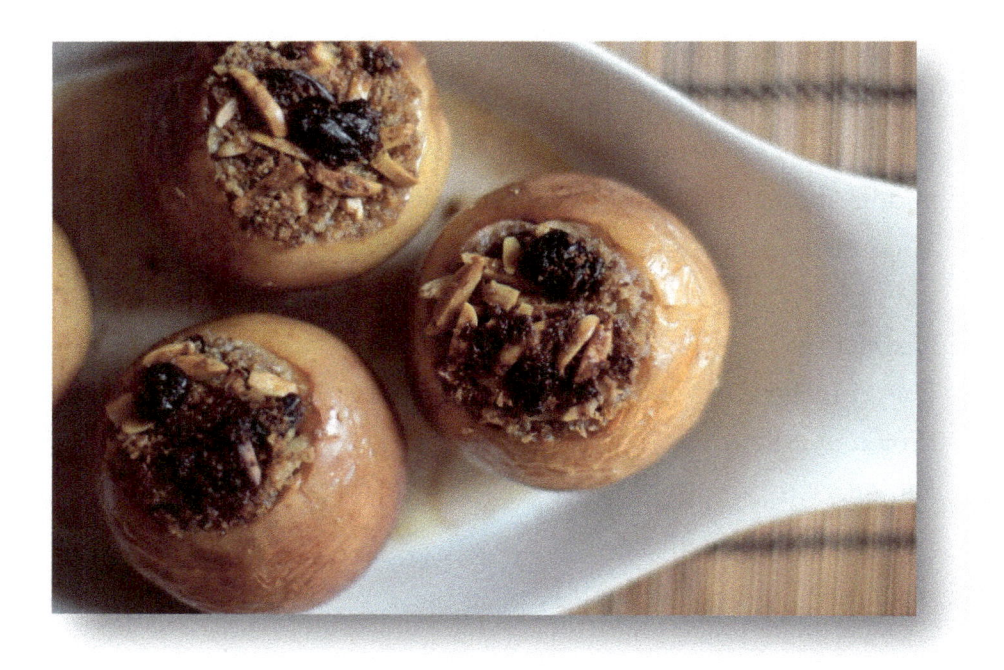

Preparation time: 15 minutes
Cooking time: 10 minutes
Servings: 4

Ingredients:
- 2 tbsp. Brown Sugar
- Four pcs. Apples
- 40 grams of mixed seeds
- 50 grams Fresh Breadcrumbs
- Zest of orange and olive oil
- 1 tsp. Mixed spice or cinnamon

Directions:

Core the apples and score skin around using a sharp knife to prevent splitting.

Mix all the rest of the Ingredients, carefully stuff the inside of the apples, and spread all remaining mix.

Bake the apple at 180° for 10 minutes until the sugar caramelized.

Nutrition:

Energy (calories): 180 kcal

Protein: 2.58 g

Fat: 5.46 g

Carbohydrates: 33.97 g

Blackberry – Apricot Crumble

Preparation time: 10 minutes
Cooking time: 10 minutes
Servings: 6-10

Ingredients:
- 1 cup of flour with a dash of salt
- 18 oz. Fresh apricots
- ½ cup of sugar
- 5 tbsp. Cold butter
- 2 tbsp. Lemon juice

Directions:
Divide the apricots into halves and the stones are removed. Then dice these and put them in a bowl. Add in the blackberries with 2 tbsp. Of sugar, mix with lemon juice and blend .
Scoop the fruit mixture into the oven dish and spread it out evenly.
In a bowl, combine the flour and salt with the remaining sugar and add the butter and one tbsp. Of cold water. Using your hands, mix these with your hand to create a crumb mixture.
Preheat the air fryer at the temperature of 390 degrees Fahrenheit.
Lay the crumbly mixture evenly on top of the fruit mixture and press down lightly.
Place the dish into the basket and put it in the air fryer, and bake for 20 minutes or until the crumble turns into golden brown and the inside well was done. You can always test by picking it with a

toothpick. If the flour no longer sticks to the toothpick, then it's cooked.

Nutrition:
Energy (calories): 214 kcal
Protein: 1.38 g
Fat: 9.84 g
Carbohydrates: 32.46 g

French Toast with Berries

Preparation time: 5 minutes
Cooking time: 5 minutes
Servings: 2

Ingredients:
- 1 tsp. Vanilla extract
- Mixed Berries Spread with a squeeze of maple syrup
- Two slices of bread (Thick)

Directions:
Spread mixed berries spread on top of the bread.
Put in the basket of the air fryer and cook over 180 degrees F for 5 minutes. Serve toast with toppings of your choice.

Nutrition:
Energy (calories): 59 kcal
Protein: 1.77 g
Fat: 0.67 g
Carbohydrates: 10.15 g

Peanut Butter – Marshmallow Turnovers

Preparation time: 10 minutes
Cooking time: 5 minutes
Servings: 4

Ingredients:

- 4 tbsp. Peanut butter
- 4 tbsp. Marshmallow fluff
- Four sheets of Filo pastry, defrosted
- 2 oz. Butter, melted
- 1 Pinch of sea salt

Directions:

Preheat the air fryer to 360 degrees Fahrenheit, then brush butter over one sheet of Filo pastry. Lay another Filo sheet on top and again, brush it with butter. Repeat the process for all of the remaining two pastry sheets.

Cut layers of Filo sheets into 4 pcs. of 3x12-inch strips

On the underside of a Filo strip, put 1 tbsp. of peanut butter and 1 tbsp. marshmallow fluff. Fold the sheet's tip to cover the filling while forming a triangular shape and fold the edges in a zigzag manner until the filling is fully wrapped inside. Use a touch of butter to seal the end of the turnover.

Place these turnovers in the cooking basket and cook in the air fryer for 3-5 minutes or until these turn golden brown and puffy.

Finish with a pinch of sea salt for a mixture of sweet and salty flavour.

Nutrition:
Energy (calories): 171 kcal
Protein: 1.94 g
Fat: 12.15 g
Carbohydrates: 14.47 g

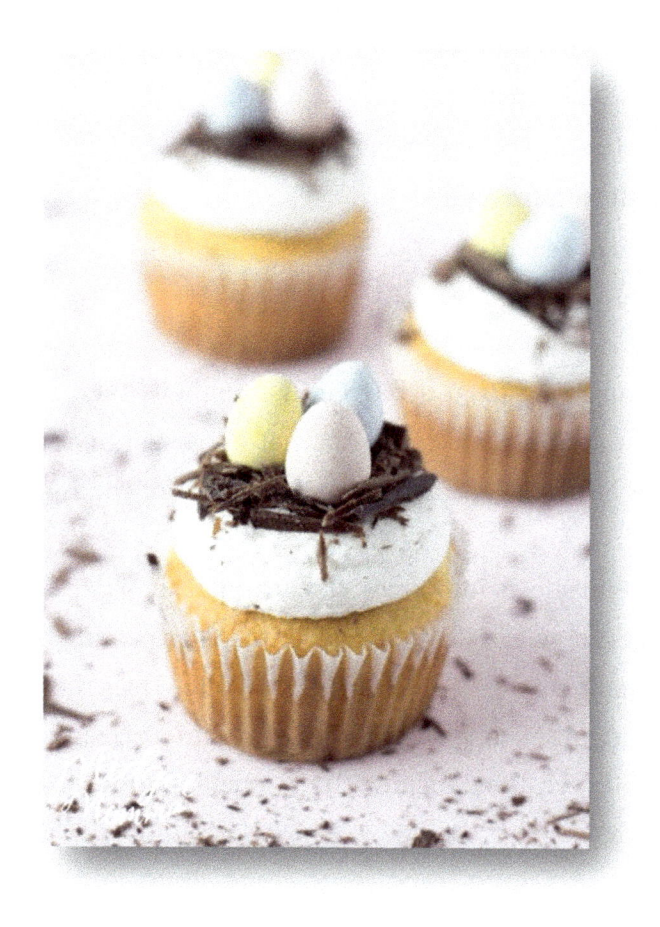

Pigs in a Blanket

Preparation time: 20 minutes
Cooking time: 15 minutes
Servings: 7

Ingredients:
- 1 -8oz can crescent dough
- 20 Vegan franks (Smart Dogs meatless hot dog)
- ¼ cup Dijon mustard
- ¼ cup of silken tofu
- Sesame seeds

Directions:
Preheat air fryer to 330 degrees F.
Cut crescent rolls dough into three equal parts, making three strips from each roll. Brush with Dijon mustard each dough strips and place the vegan hotdogs on one end of the dough and roll it up.
Arrange these on the fryer and cook for approximately 8 minutes. Move the temperature up to 390 degrees F and cook for another 3 minutes or until they turn golden brown.

Nutrition:
Energy (calories): 76 kcal
Protein: 2.7 g
Fat: 2.58 g
Carbohydrates: 10.36 g

Toasted Bread Sandwich

Preparation time: 5 minutes
Cooking time: 6 minutes
Servings: 4

Ingredients:
- 1 English muffin
- Salt and pepper to taste

Directions:
Place the muffin inside the air fryer.

Heat the air fryer to 200 degrees Centigrade or 395 degrees Fahrenheit for about 6 minutes.

Arrange the sandwich and serve. Stuff your sandwich with any desired fillings.

Nutrition:
Energy (calories): 68 kcal
Fat: 0.59 g
Carbohydrates: 13.83 g

Banana Bread Pudding

Preparation time: 10 minutes
Cooking time: 50 minutes
Servings: 4

Ingredients

- One 16-ounce loaf of French bread
- ½ cup raisins
- 1 ½ cup of unsweetened almond milk vanilla or plain (or other non-dairy milk)
- 1 cup mashed overripe bananas
- ¼ cup maple syrup
- ¼ cup dark brown sugar
- 2 tsp. cornstarch or potato starch
- 2 tsp. vanilla extract
- 1 ½ tsp. cinnamon
- ½ tsp. baking powder
- ½ tsp. nutmeg
- ¼ tsp. allspice
- Sauce
- ½ cup apple cider or apple juice
- ¼ cup maple syrup
- 1 tsp. cornstarch mixed with 1 tbsp. apple juice
- 1 ½ - 2 tbsp. brandy, rum, or bourbon (see Notes below)
- ¼ cup chopped pecans or walnuts optional

Directions:

Break the bread or tear it into bits that are bite-sized. Spread it out on a cookie sheet if the bread looks sticky or dense and toast it in the oven for a few minutes. Place it and put the raisins in a large bowl.

In the blender, mix non-dairy milk with banana, maple syrup, sugar, cornstarch, vanilla, baking powder and spices. Blend until perfectly smooth. Spill it over the bread using a silicon spatula. Stir well to cover all of the bread thoroughly. Put aside for a few minutes to soak while you are cleaning the pan and preheating the oven.

Preheat the furnace to 350F. Using parchment paper or foil to cover an 8 to 8-inch baking dish thinly. Pour the bread pudding in an even layer into the tub. Bake for 45 minutes or until the top is set and begins to brown. Take it out of the oven and let it cool for at least 15 minutes.

Make the sauce while the pudding is cooling. In a small saucepan, put the apple cider and maple syrup over medium heat and bring to a simmer, sometimes stirring, until approximately half the volume is reduced. Add the cornstarch mixture carefully and stir constantly, bring it to a boil, and simmer for a few more minutes until the mixture is no longer cloudy.

Remove from the heat and add a little at a time, to sample the brandy or other spirits. Stir the nuts in. Poke a few holes with a toothpick at the top of the bread pudding and pour the sauce over the top, uniformly spreading the nuts. Slice into squares, then serve.

Nutrition:

Energy (calories): 631 kcal

Protein: 14.44 g

Fat: 7.59 g
Carbohydrates: 126.59 g

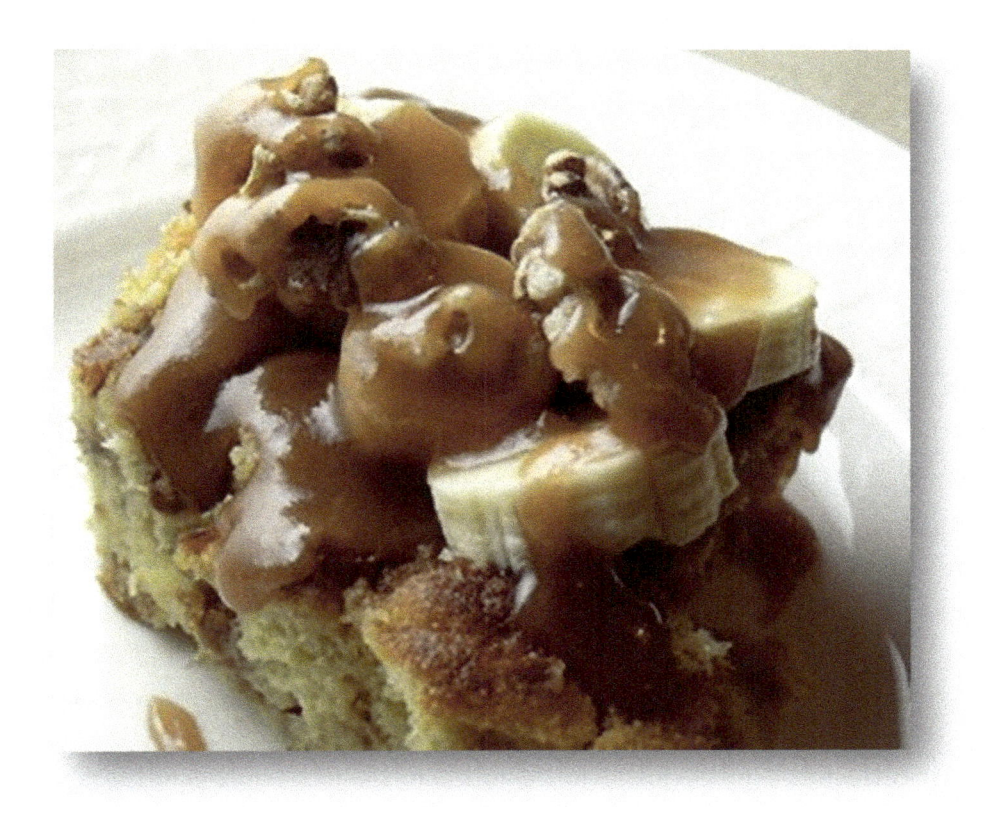

Apple Cinnamon Scuffins

Preparation time: 10 minutes
Cooking time: 15 minutes
Servings: 4

Ingredients:
- 2 cups oat flour
- 1 tsp. baking powder
- 1 cup rolled oats
- ½ tsp. baking soda
- ¼ tsp. salt
- 1 tsp. cinnamon powder
- ½ cup date paste
- ½ cup currants
- ½ cup dairy-free yogurt
- ½ cup almond milk
- ½ cups chopped red apples
- Confectioner's sugar for sprinkling

Directions:

In a prepared bowl, combine all the dry Ingredients. Then, in another bowl, mix the date paste, dairy-free yogurt, and almond milk.

Add the cinnamon mixture to the milk mixture and combine. After, fold in the apples.

In baking sheet that can fit into the air fryer, line with parchment paper, and drop large spoonful's of the batter on the sheet.

Sprinkle with confectioner's sugar and bake at 350 F for 12 to 15 minutes.

Remove when ready, allow cooling, and serve.

Nutrition:

Calories 105

Total Fat 1g

Total Carbs 15g

Fibre 4g

Net Carbs 11g

Protein 9g

Custard and Rhubarb Pie

Preparation time: 15 minutes
Cooking time: 38 minutes
Servings: 4

Ingredients:
- One pie shell, unbaked
- 3 cups rhubarb, cut into small pieces
- 1 cup coconut cream
- 4 tbsp aquafaba, whisked
- One ¼ cup sugar
- 2 tbsp. flour
- ½ tsp. salt

Directions:
Unwrap the pie shell and place the rhubarb in the crust. The pie shell's size should fit into your fryer basket.

In a bowl, whisk the remaining Ingredients until properly combined and pour into the crust.

Preheat the air fryer.

Put the cake into the fryer basket and bake at 400 F for 8 minutes, then reduce the temperature to 350 F degrees and cook further for 30 minutes or until the custard sets but is fluffy in the middle.

Remove the pie, allow cooling, slice, and serve.

Nutrition:

Calories 215

Total Fat 10g

Total Carbs 28g

Fibre 3g

Net Carbs 25g

Protein 3g

Vegan Snacks

Avocado Rolls

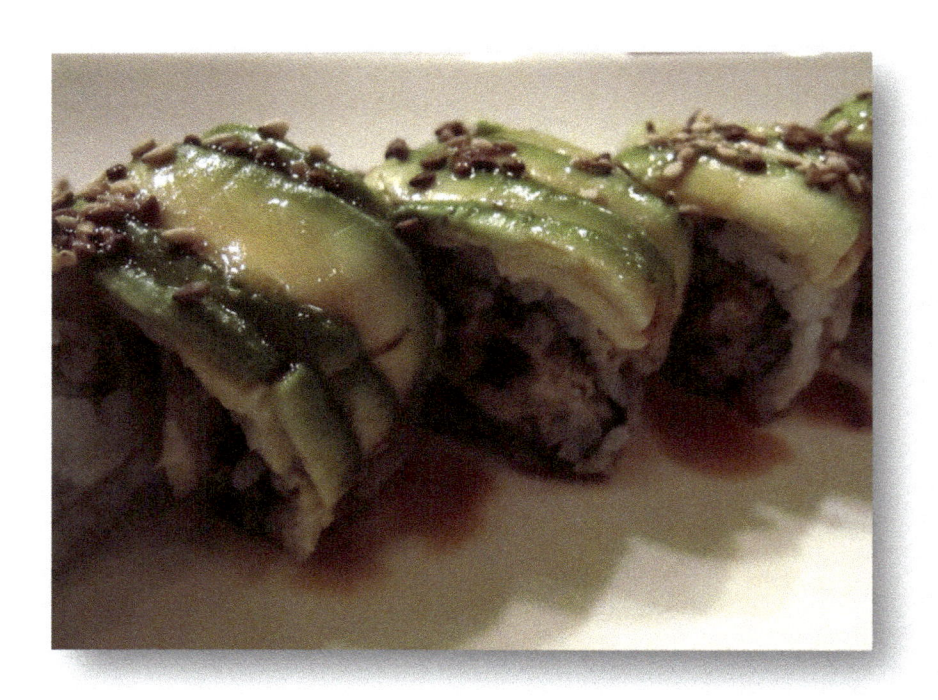

Preparation time: 20 minutes
Cooking time: 25 minutes
Servings: 5

Ingredients:
- Ten rice paper wrappers

- Three avocados, sliced
- One tomato, diced
- Salt and pepper to taste
- 1 tbsp. olive oil
- 4 tbsp. sriracha
- 2 tbsp. sugar
- 1 tbsp. rice vinegar
- 1 tbsp. sesame oil

Directions:
Mash avocados in a bowl.
Stir in the tomatoes, salt and pepper.
Mix well.
Arrange the rice paper wrappers.
Scoop mixture on top.
Roll and seal the edges with water.
Cook in the air fryer at 350 degrees F for 5 minutes.
Mix the rest of the Ingredients.
Serve rolls with the sriracha dipping sauce.

Nutrition:
Calories 422
Saturated Fat 5.8g
Total Carbohydrate 38.7g
Dietary Fiber 8.8g
Protein 3.8g
Potassium 633mg

Fried Ravioli

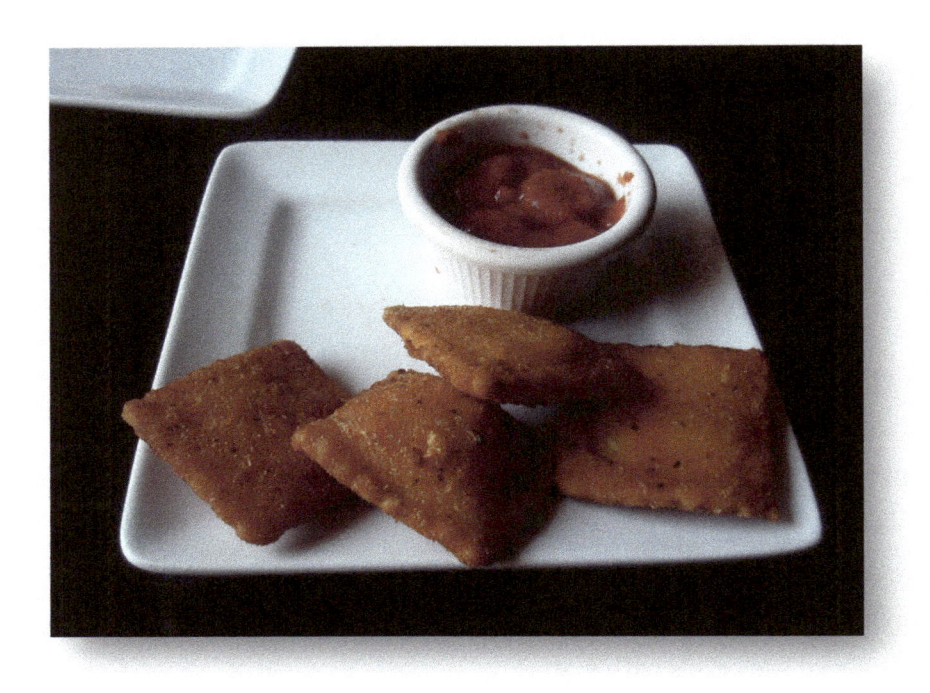

Preparation time: 15 minutes
Cooking time: 8 minutes
Servings: 4

Ingredients:
- ½ cup panko breadcrumbs
- Salt and pepper to taste
- 1 tsp. garlic powder
- 1 tsp. dried oregano
- 1 tsp. dried basil

- 2 tsp. Nutritional yeast flakes
- ¼ cup aquafaba liquid
- 8 oz. frozen vegan ravioli
- Cooking spray
- ½ cup marinara sauce

Directions:

Mix the breadcrumbs, salt, pepper, garlic powder, oregano, basil and Nutritional yeast flakes on a plate.

In another bowl, pour the aquafaba liquid.

Dip each ravioli into the liquid and then coat it with the breadcrumb mixture.

Put the ravioli in the air fryer.

Spray oil on the ravioli.

Cook at 390 degrees F for 6 minutes.

Flip each one and cook for another 2 minutes.

Serve with marinara sauce.

Nutrition:

Calories 154

Total Fat 3.8g

Saturated Fat 0.6g

Total Carbohydrate 18.4g

Dietary Fiber 1.5g

Protein 4.6g

Potassium 154mg

Corn Fritters

Preparation time: 15 minutes
Cooking time: 10 minutes
Servings: 4

Ingredients:
- ¼ cup ground cornmeal
- ¼ cup flour
- Salt and pepper to taste
- ½ tsp. baking powder
- ¼ tsp. garlic powder
- ¼ tsp. onion powder
- ¼ tsp. paprika
- ¼ cup parsley, chopped
- One cup corn kernels mixed with 3 tbsp. almond milk
- 2 cups fresh corn kernels
- 4 tbsp. vegan mayonnaise
- 2 tsp. grainy mustard

Directions:
Mix the cornmeal, flour, salt, pepper, baking powder, garlic powder, onion powder, paprika and parsley in a bowl.
Put the corn kernels with almond milk in a food processor.
Season with salt and pepper.
Pulse until well blended.

Add the corn kernels.

Transfer to a bowl and stir into the cornmeal mixture.

Pour a small amount of the batter into the air fryer pan.

Pour another a few centimetres away from the first cake.

Cook in the air fryer set the temperature at 350 degrees for 10 minutes or until golden.

Flip halfway through.

Serve with mayo mustard dip.

Nutrition:

Calories 135

Total Fat 4.6g

Saturated Fat 0.2g

Cholesterol 0mg

Sodium 136mg

Total Carbohydrate 22.5g

Dietary Fiber 2.5g

Total Sugars 2.7g

Protein 3.5g

Potassium 308mg

Mushroom Pizza

Preparation time: 15 minutes
Cooking time: 10 minutes
Servings: 4

Ingredients:
- Four large Portobello mushrooms, stems and gills removed
- 1 tsp. balsamic vinegar
- Salt and pepper to taste
- 4 tbsp. vegan pasta sauce
- One clove garlic, minced
- 3 oz. zucchini, chopped
- Four olives, sliced
- 2 tbsp. sweet red pepper, diced
- 1 tsp. dried basil
- ½ cups hummus
- Fresh basil, minced

Directions:
Coat the mushrooms with balsamic vinegar and season with salt and pepper.
Spread pasta sauce inside each mushroom.
Sprinkle with minced garlic.
Preheat your air fryer to 330 degrees F.
Cook mushrooms for 3 minutes.
Take the mushrooms out and top with zucchini, olives, and peppers.

Season with salt, pepper and basil.

Put them back in the air fryer and cook for another 3 minutes.

Serve mushroom pizza with hummus and fresh basil.

Nutrition:

Calories 70

Total Fat 1.56 g

Total Carbohydrate 11 g

Dietary Fiber 3.4 g

Protein 4.3 g

Vegan Bread and Pizza

Whole Wheat Vegan Toast

Preparation time: 5 minutes
Cooking time: 10 minutes
Servings: 3

Ingredients:

- 1 Loaf of sliced whole wheat bread
- 2 Ripe bananas
- 1 Can of coconut milk
- 2 Tsp. of vanilla
- 1 Tsp. of cinnamon
- ¼ Tsp. of salt
- ½ Cup of dry roasted pecans
- Cooking spray

Directions:

Start by cutting the whole-wheat bread into equal-sized slices

In a blender, mix the coconut milk, the pecan, the vanilla, the cinnamon, and the salt. Pour your obtained mixture into a deep bowl; then add the bread and let soak for about 2 minutes

Grease a baking tray and preheat your air fryer to about 350° F

Lay the soaked bread into the greased tray and put it in the basket of the air fryer

Close the lid and then set the timer to about 8 minutes and the temperature to 360°F

When the timer beeps, remove the bread toasts from the air fryer; then set it aside to cool for about 5 minutes

Serve and enjoy with maple syrup!

Note:

This whole wheat Vegan French toast is very decadent, creamy. Try it and enjoy the warmth. This recipe will make you addicted to it with its light taste. You can earn top this vegan toast with any topping of your choice.

Nutrition:

Calories per serving 110 calories

Fat per serving 0.9 grams

Saturated Fats 0.2 gram

Total Carbs per serving 21.1 grams

Protein per serving 4 grams

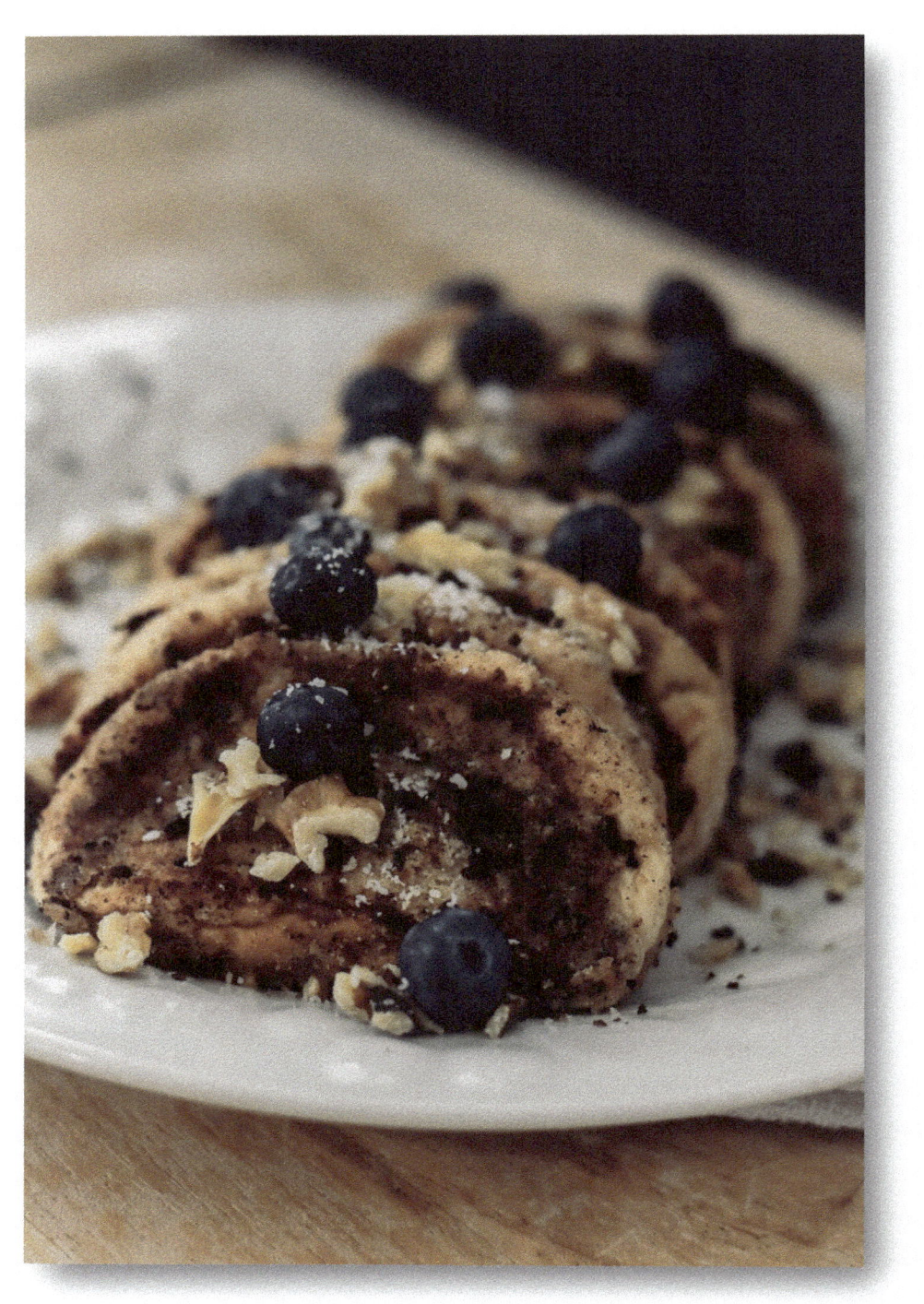

Flat Bread with Olive and Rosemary

Preparation time: 15 minutes
Cooking time: 20 minutes
Servings: 5
Note:
With the crispiness of the pizza crust and the delicious taste of the pita bread, this recipe will offer you a magical combination of both types. This recipe is light and topped with spices; you will like it.

Ingredients:

- One and ½ tsp. of active dry yeast
- One and ½ tsp. of unrefined cane sugar
- ½ Tsp. of kosher salt
- One and ½ cups of all-purpose flour
- One and ½ cups of whole spelt flour
- 1 Tbsp. of finely cut fresh rosemary leaves
- 2 Tbsp. of extra-virgin olive oil
- 2 Tbsp. of thyme
- ½ Cup of pitted and cut olive

Directions:

In a deep mixing bowl, mix a little bit of olive oil with a little bit of yeast, salt, sugar and pour in about 1 cup of water (Make sure the water is warm)

Set aside the mixture and let rest for about 11 minutes

Add in the flours and the chopped rosemary; then blend the Ingredients on a deficient speed

Use the dough hook to knead your dough, and once you obtain a smooth one; divide it into about two balls

Put the dough balls over a floured baking paper and let rest for about 3 hour s

Put the pizza over a greased baking tray and use your hands and fingers to spread it into a circle

Cover your bread with a kitchen towel and set it aside to rest for about 12 minutes

Brush the bread with olive oil and put it in the basket of the air fryer; close the lid and set the timer to about 10 minutes and the temperature to about 365° F

When the timer beeps, remove the bread from the air fryer and sprinkle a little bit of pepper, olive oil and salt

Serve and enjoy!

Nutrition:

Calories per serving – 156.4 calories

Fat per serving – 10.1 grams

Saturated Fats – 2.5 gram

Total Carbs per serving – 4.6 grams

Protein per serving – 6.1 grams

Cinnamon Sugar Toast

Preparation time: 10 minutes
Cooking time: 8 minutes
Servings: 2

Ingredients:
- 1/4 cup granulated sugar
- 11/2 tsp. ground cinnamon
- 2 tbsp. vegan butter, room temperature
- 4 slices gluten-free sandwich bread

Directions:
In a prepared small bowl, combine sugar and cinnamon.
Preheat the air fryer set the temperature at 375°F for 3 minutes.
Spread butter over bread slices. Evenly sprinkle buttered slices with cinnamon-sugar mix.
Place two bread slices in an ungreased air fryer basket and cook for 4 minutes. Transfer to a large plate. Repeat with remaining pieces. Serve warm.

Nutrition:
Energy (calories): 193 kcal
Protein: 5.68 g
Fat: 7.54 g
Carbohydrates: 26.89 g

Salted Caramel Banana Muffins

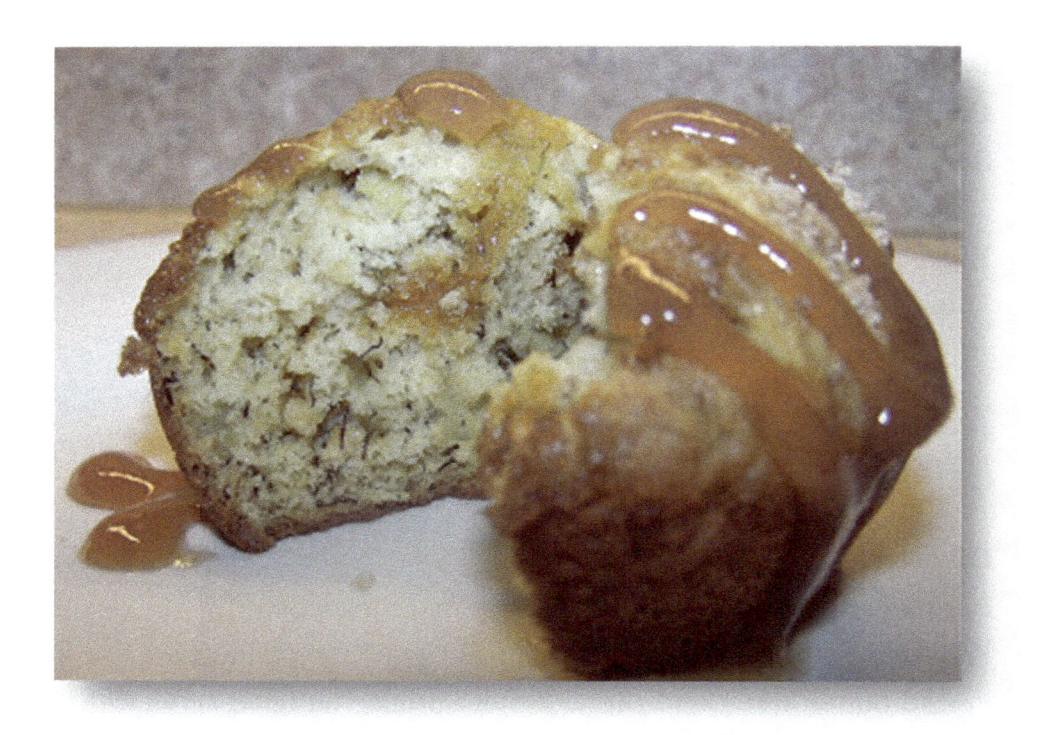

Preparation time: 10 minutes
Cooking time: 14 minutes
Servings: 8

Ingredients:
- 1 cup gluten-free all-purpose flour
- 1/2 tsp. baking soda
- 1/3 cup granulated sugar
- 1/4 tsp. salt

- 1/3 cup mashed banana, about one large ripe banana
- 1/2 tsp. vanilla extract
- 1 Silken tofu
- 1 tbsp. vegetable oil
- 1/4 cup salted caramel chips

Directions:

Preheat the air fryer set the temperature at 375°F for 3 minutes.

In a prepared large mixing bowl, combine flour, baking soda, sugar, and salt. In a separate prepared medium bowl, combine mashed banana, vanilla, tofu, and oil.

Pour all wet Ingredients into dry Ingredients and gently combine. Fold in salted caramel chips. Do not overmix. Spoon mixture into eight silicone cupcake liners lightly greased with preferred cooking oil.

Place four muffins in an air fryer basket. Cook for 7 minutes, then transfer to a cooling rack. Repeat with remaining muffins. Serve warm or cooled.

Nutrition:

Energy (calories): 103 kcal

Protein: 1.77 g

Fat: 1.93 g

Carbohydrates: 19.71 g

Pizza Tofu Bites

These little bites of tasty protein are perfect for an after-school treat or a snack on the weekend. Marinating the tofu helps it soak up the flavours before air frying. Dipping the bites into a bowl of warmed marinara sauce will bring all the ingredients together.

Preparation time: 15 minutes
Cooking time: 20 minutes
Servings: 4

Ingredients:
- For Marinade
- 1/3 cup vegetable broth
- 2 tbsp. tomato sauce
- 1 tbsp. Nutritional yeast
- 1 tsp. Italian seasoning
- 1 tsp. granulated sugar
- 1/2 tsp. fennel seeds
- 1/2 tsp. garlic powder
- 1/4 tsp. salt
- 1/4 tsp. ground black pepper
- 14 oz firm tofu, cut into 3/4" cubes
- For Breading
- 2/3 cup plain gluten-free bread crumbs
- 2 tsp. Nutritional yeast

- 1 tsp. Italian seasoning
- 1/2 tsp. salt
- For Dip
- 1 cup marinara sauce, heated

Directions:

To Make the marinade: Combine all Marinade Ingredients in a gallon-sized plastic bag or large bowl. Toss tofu to coat. Refrigerate for 30 minutes, tossing tofu once more after 15 minutes.

To make Breading and Pizza Tofu Bites: Preheat air fryer to 350°F for 3 minutes.

In a shallow dish, combine Breading Ingredients.

Strain marinade from tofu cubes. Dredge in bread crumb mixture.

Place half of the tofu in an air fryer basket lightly greased with preferred cooking oil. Cook 5 minutes. Flip tofu. Brush with additional cooking oil—Cook an additional 5 minutes.

Transfer cooked tofu to a large plate. Repeat with remaining tofu. Serve warm with marinara dip on the side.

Nutrition:

Energy (calories): 422 kcal

Fat: 27.84 g

Carbohydrates: 26.85 g

Vegan Main Dishes

The Great Taquito

"Refried beans and a mixture of creamy delight packed in a tortilla, these taquitos are Vegan and Guilt-free!"

Preparation time: 15 minutes
Cooking time: 15 minutes
Servings: 4
Temperature: 392degreesF
Prep Time: 5 minutes
Cook Time: 7 minutes

Ingredients:
- Eight corn tortillas
- Cooking oil spray as needed
- 1 (15 ounces) can vegan refried beans
- 1 cup shredded vegan cheese
- Guacamole
- Cashew cheese
- Vegan sour cream
- Fresh salsa

Directions:

Preheat your Air Fryer to 392 degrees F

Warm your tortilla and run them underwater for a second, transfer to Air Fryer cooking basket and cook for 1 minute

Remove to the flat surface and place equal amounts of beans at the center of each tortilla, top with vegan cheese

Roll tortilla sides up over filling, place seam side down in Air Fryer

Spray oil on top and cook for 7 minutes until golden brown

Serve and enjoy!

Nutrition:

Calories: 420

Fat: 5g

Carbohoydrates: 80g

Protein: 15g

The Cheesy Vegan Sandwich

Preparation time: 3 minutes
Cooking time: 12 minutes
Servings: 4
Temperature: 392degreesF

Ingredients:
- Two slices sprouted whole grain bread
- 1 tsp. vegan margarine
- Two slices of vegan chees e
- 1 tsp. mellow white miso
- One medium-large garlic clove, minced
- 2 tbsp. fermented vegetables, kimchi or sauerkraut
- Romaine lettuce

Directions:
Preheat your Air Fryer to 392 degrees F
Spread outside of bread with Vegan margarine, place sliced cheese inside and close sandwich back up
Transfer Sandwich to Air Fryer and cook 6 minutes, flip and cook for 6 minutes more
Transfer to plate and spread miso and garlic clove inside one of the slices, top with fermented veggies and lettuce
Close sandwich and cut in half
Serve and enjoy!

Nutrition:

Calories: 288

Fat: 13g

Carbohoydrates: 34g

Protein: 8g

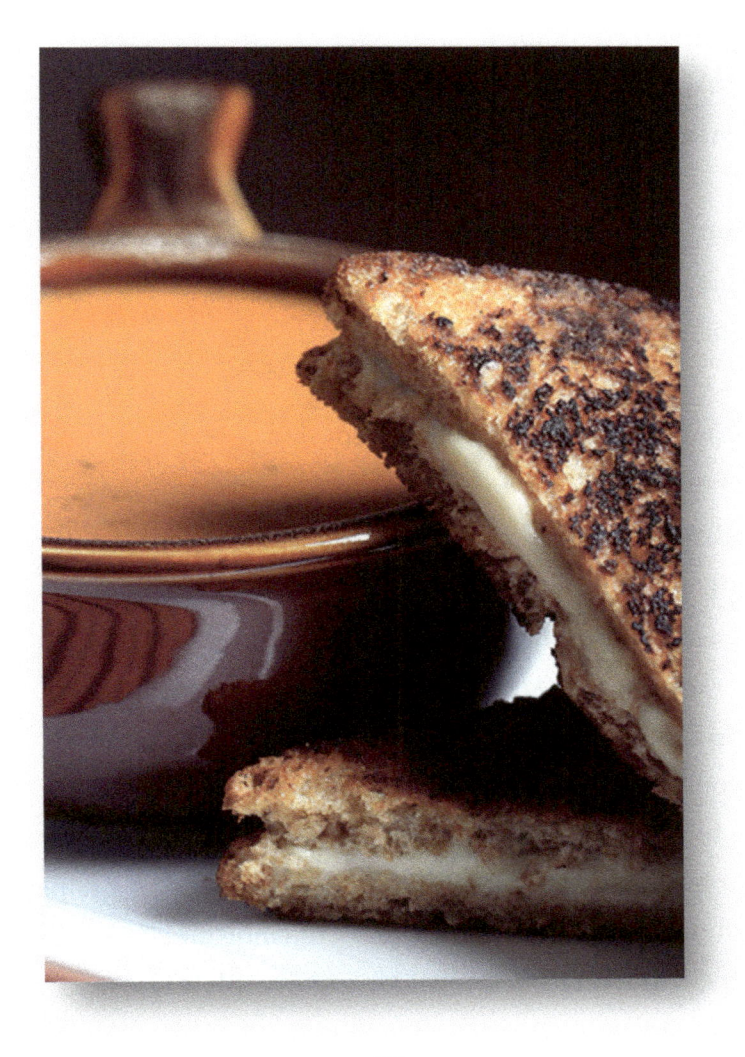

Sesame Crunchy Tofu

"Sesame dressed crunchy tofu! This is the vegan protein dish to beat!"

Preparation time: 10 minutes
Cooking time: 20 minutes
Servings: 4
Temperature: 392degreesF

Ingredients:
- One pack (8 ounces) tofu, extra firm
- One and ½ tbsp. tamari
- ½ tsp. granulated garlic
- ½ cup sesame seeds, raw and toasted
- 2 tsp. flour
- 1 tbsp. arrowroot
- 2 tbsp. sunflower oil
- Cooking oil spray as needed

Directions:
Preheat your Air Fryer to 392 degrees F
Slice tofu into ½ inch thick slabs, then into triangles
Press tofu by placing the pieces in a fine layer on top of a paper towel, cover with more towels and gently press the moisture
Place pressed tofu on a plate, sprinkle evenly with tamari and garlic
Turn to coat well

Take a medium bowl; add sesame seeds, flour, and arrowroot

Add tofu and stir well, coat with sesame mixture

Add oil and stir to coat the tofu

Spray Air Fryer basket with oil, transfer tofu to a single layer and bake for 10 minutes

Remove, turn the pieces and cook for 10 minutes more until golden brown and crisp

Serve and enjoy!

Nutrition:
Calories: 183
Fat: 18g
Carbohoydrates: 5g
Protein: 4g

Vegan Staples

Korean Fried Tempeh

Spicy and slightly sweet, these utterly delicious and vegan Korean fried tempeh are perfect as they have no added oil. They're full of protein, lower in fat and an ideal appetizer served with white rice and veggies as a main course.

Preparation time: 10 minutes
Cooking time: 20 minutes
Servings: 2-4

Ingredients:
- For the Tempeh:
- 200g tempeh, cut into medium-sized chunks
- 3 - 4 tbsp. Panko breadcrumbs
- 2 tbsp. vegan mayonnaise
- For the Sauce:
- 2 tbsp. Gochujang Korean red chilli paste
- 1 tbsp. maple or agave syrup
- Two cloves garlic, minced
- 1tbsp. water
- 1 tbsp. soy sauce
- Salt and pepper, to taste

- To Serve:
- 1 tbsp. sesame seeds
- 1 tsp. fresh chopped chives
- Chive flowers (optional)

Directions:

To make the breaded tempeh, plate the vegan mayo and breadcrumbs into separate shallow bowls.

Mix few drops of water with the mayo to thin it out.

Dip each piece of tempeh in mayo and then in the breadcrumbs and place into the air fryer basket.

Cook the tempeh in the air fryer for 15 minutes, flipping the pieces over every 4-5 minutes until they becomes golden brown and crispy.

When the tempeh is just about cooked, add the sauce to a frying pan, mix to form a paste and cook on medium heat for 2 - 3 minutes until slightly thick, glossy and bubbling.

Add the breaded tempeh and stir gently until fully coated.

Garnish with the chives and sesame seeds, then serve as a snack or with white rice and veggies of your choice.

Nutrition:

Energy (calories): 235 kcal

Protein: 14.96 g

Fat: 13.8 g

Carbohydrates: 17.48 g

Lemon Tofu Piccata

Preparation time: 30 minutes
Cooking time: 20 minutes
Servings: 4

Ingredients:
- For the Marinade:
- ¼ cup fresh lemon juic e
- One clove garlic, minced
- 2 tbsp. parsley
- ½ tsp. black pepper
- ½ tsp. sea salt
- For the Tofu:
- One block extra-firm tofu, cut into eight rectangular cutlets
- 1 cup Panko breadcrumbs or vegan breadcrumbs
- ½ cup vegan mayo
- For the Sauce:
- ¼ cup lemon juice
- 1 cup vegetable broth
- 2 tbsp. fresh parsley
- One clove garlic, minced
- 2 tsp. potato starch or cornstarch
- 2 tbsp. capers
- ¼ tsp. black pepper
- ½ tsp. sea salt

- To Serve:
- One lemon, sliced into rounds

Directions:

To marinate the Tofu:

Mix all the marinade Ingredients in a blender or food processor.

Puree to a pretty smooth mix. In a prepared shallow bowl or on a large plate, cover the tofu with the marinade and marinate for 15-30 minutes

To bread the Tofu:

Put the vegan mayo into a shallow bowl and the Panko breadcrumbs in another shallow bowl.

Dredge each tofu cutlet first in the mayo, then in the breadcrumbs, making sure to get an even coating.

To cook the Tofu:

Arrange the tofu cutlets in a single layer in the air fryer basket. Cook in batches at degrees, Fahrenheit for 20 minutes, shaking the cutlets gently after 10 minutes to prevent sticking.

Repeat in batches, if needed.

To make the Lemon Piccata Sauce:

While the tofu cooks, put all together the sauce Ingredients, except the capers in a blender or food processor.

Puree until smooth, and then stir in the capers.

Pour the sauce into a small saucepan.

Let it boil and then reduce to a simmer, stirring for 5-7 minutes, until it thickens.

Serve:

Spoon a couple of tbsp. Of the sauce over the breaded tofu cutlets and garnish with the lemon and parsley.

Nutrition:

Energy (calories): 694 kcal

Protein: 11.95 g

Fat: 71.2 g

Carbohydrates: 10.27 g

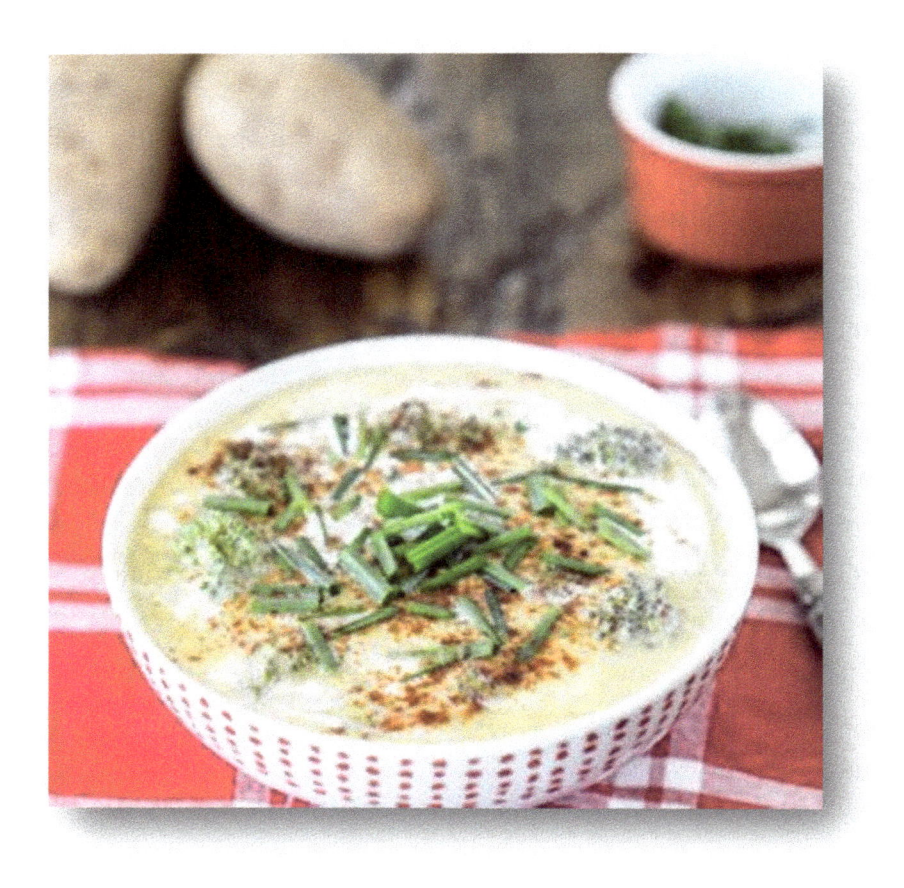

Bbq Lentil Meatballs

These air fryer BBQ Lentil Meatballs are flavorful and chewy on the inside and satisfyingly crunchy on the outside. They're merely addictive served with your favourite vegan BBQ sauce.

Preparation time: 5 minutes
Cooking time: 40 minutes
Servings: 2

Ingredients:
- For the Lentil Meatballs:
- 2 cups vegetable stock
- 1 cup dry brown or green lentils
- ½ cup chopped dried mushrooms
- 2 tbsp. sunflower oil
- 1 cup white or yellow onion, finely diced
- 1 tbsp. tomato paste
- One clove garlic, minced
- 3 tbsp. vegan BBQ sauce
- ½ cup wheat gluten
- 2 tbsp. water or vegetable stock
- 1 tbsp. Vegan Worcestershire or low-sodium soy sauce
- ½ tsp. smoked paprika
- 1 tsp. onion powder
- 1 tsp. Dried parsley

- ¼ tsp. Black pepper
- ½ tsp. salt to taste
- For the Topping:
- 1 cup vegan BBQ sauce

Directions:

Over medium-high heat, a large pot brings the vegetable stock, lentils, and mushrooms to a boil. Adjust heat lower and simmer for 20 minutes, until the lentils are tender and the liquid absorbed.

In a small pan, warm the oil over medium heat. Add the onions and sauté for 7 - 10 minutes, or until onions are just beginning to caramelize.

Next, adjust the heat to a medium-low and add the tomato paste and garlic. Sauté for another minute or so, and then set the pan aside.

In a food processor, place cooked lentil-mushrooms mixture, onion-tomato mixture, wheat gluten, vegan Bbq sauce, water, Worcestershire sauce, onion powder, parsley, smoked paprika, salt and pepper. Pulse until the mixture is well combined but still chunky.

Coat the air fryer basket with a light spray of cooking oil.

Moisten clean hands with water, then form roughly 2-tbsp. Worth of the mixture into lentil balls.

Put each ball inside the air fryer basket, leaving at least half an inch between them.

Coat the lentil balls with a light spray of cooking oil and cook at 350 degrees Fahrenheit for 12 minutes. Transfer the lentil meatballs to a plate or platter, then drizzle the vegan BBQ sauce over the top

Serve immediately with toothpicks, and enjoy!

Nutrition:

Energy (calories): 2172 kcal

Protein: 8.37 g

Fat: 237.43 g

Carbohydrates: 27.22 g

Cajun French fry Po'boy with Vegan Mushroom Gravy

This New Orleans features crispy French fries sandwiched inside of a baguette and smothered with gravy. This vegan version is also good and utterly delicious!

Preparation time: 20 minutes
Cooking time: 15 minutes
Servings: 4

Ingredients:
- For the French fries:
- Four medium Russet potatoes, cut in half, and then into planks
- 6 cups of boiling water for soaking the potatoes
- 2 tsp. olive oil (or use aquafaba)
- 1 tsp. Cajun seasoning
- ¼ tsp. granulated garlic
- ½ tsp. smoked paprika
- ¼ tsp. ground black pepper
- ½ tsp. salt
- Mushroom Gravy Ingredients:
- 1 tbsp. olive oil (use water if the recipe is oil-free)
- 3 cups chopped mushrooms
- 2 tsp. vegan Worcestershire sauce
- 2 tsp. soy sauce (you may substitute for coconut aminos)

- 1 tbsp. tapioca starch
- ½ cup of water
- To Serve:
- French or Italian soft loaf
- Lettuce
- Sliced tomatoes
- Vegan mayo
- Favourite hot sauce

Directions:

To make the French Fries:

Place the fries in a bowl or saucepan.

Let the water boil and then pour over the fries, covering them.

Soak the potatoes in hot water for 15 minutes, and then drain over the sink.

Once dry, toss the fries in the oil (or aquafaba if using), paprika, garlic, Cajun seasoning, salt and black pepper.

Add the fries to the air fryer basket and cook at 350 degrees Fahrenheit for 5 minutes. Shake the basket and cook further for 5 minutes.

Raise the heat to 390 degrees Fahrenheit and cook for another 5 minutes.

Shake the basket and then cook a final 5 minutes.

To make the Mushroom Gravy:

While the potatoes are in the air fryer, heat 1 tbsp. Olive oil in a prepared large skillet over medium heat.

Add the mushrooms and sauté until they begin to release all their juices.

Stir in the Worcestershire sauce and soy sauce and cook for 2 minutes.
Add the water and stir in the tapioca starch.
Set the heat up to medium-high and cook until the sauce is thick.
To assemble the Po'Boy:
Slice the bread in half lengthways.
Toast the bread if preferred and spread it with vegan mayo and hot sauce.
Layer the baked fries at the bottom piece of the bread. Spread the mushroom mixture on top of the fries.
Serve dressed in lettuce, tomato, and mayo. Put the top piece of bread and enjoy!

Nutrition:
Energy (calories): 381 kcal
Protein: 10.49 g
19%
Fat: 6.7 g
Carbohydrates: 73.41 g

Bbq Soy Curls

Serve them accompanied with potato salad & greens for utter deliciousness.

Preparation time: 13 minutes
Cooking time: 8 minutes
Servings: 2

Ingredients:
- 1 cup of soy curls
- 1 cup of warm water
- 1 tsp. canola oil
- 1 tsp. vegetarian stock base*
- ¼ cup vegan BBQ sauce

Directions:
Soak the soy curls in water and vegetable bouillon in a bowl for about 10 minutes.
Drain the soy curls on a sieve, and squeeze out all excess water.
Place then into a mixing bowl, and pull them apart into shreds resembling string cheese.
Air fry the soy curls at 400 degrees Fahrenheit for 3 minutes. Work in batches to prevent overcrowding and to allow the rings to crisp up properly.
Remove the soy curls put them back to the mixing bowl, toss in vegan BBQ sauce and stir.

Make sure all of the curls get coated.

Return to air fryer and cook at 400 degrees Fahrenheit for 5 minutes stopping twice to shake the pan.

Serve the curls with a vegan potato salad, mixed greens, and a non-dairy mac and cheese.

Nutrition:

Energy (calories): 102 kcal

Protein: 12.04 g

Fat: 2.69 g

Carbohydrates: 9.31 g

Buttermilk Battered Tofu

Buttermilk Battered Tofu is exceptionally delicious and utterly crispy. Serve with mashed potatoes in a salad or a sandwich.

Preparation time: 20 minutes
Cooking time: 15 minutes
Servings: 2

Ingredients:
- For the Tofu:
- 8 oz. block medium-firm tofu, cut lengthways into four slices
- ½ tsp. pepper
- 1 tsp. salt
- For the Dry Ingredients:
- 1½ cups all-purpose flour
- 1/3 cup cornstarch
- 1 tbsp. paprika
- 2 tsp. cayenne
- 1 tbsp. onion powder
- 1 tbsp. garlic powder
- 1 tbsp. salt
- For the Wet Ingredients:
- 2 tbsp. vegan egg powder, mixed with ½ cup ice cold water
- One cup soymilk, mixed with 2 tsp. apple cider vinegar
- 1 tbsp. hot sauce

- 2 tbsp. bourbon
- Cooking spray oil
- For the Sambal Mayo:
- 1 tbsp. to ¼ cup sambal
- ½ cup vegan mayo
- To Serve:
- Hamburger buns
- ¼ red onion, sliced thinly
- One jalapeño, thinly sliced
- 2 cups red or green cabbage
- Bread and butter pickles
- Vegan butter, for toasting the buns
-

Directions:

Tofu Preparation:

Place the tofu on a wire rack set inside a lined baking sheet. Season with salt and pepper and let chill for an hour.

Combine all the dry Ingredients in a prepared medium-sized bowl.

Combine all the wet Ingredients in a separate medium-sized bowl.

Coat the tofu in the dry mixture and place back onto the wire rack.

Pour 3 tablespoon of the wet mixture into the dry mixture and using your hands combine the two.

Dip the tofu into the wet mixture, then pack the moistened dry flour mixture firmly around each piece.

Place the battered tofu back on the wire rack and place it into the refrigerator to chill for 30 minutes.

Spray the tofu evenly with cooking oil spray.

Place into the air fryer set at the temperature of 400 degrees Fahrenheit and cook for 10 minutes. Flip the slabs over halfway through cooking.

Add a little more spray over any areas that look dry and cook for an additional minute or two if needed.

The tofu should be a deep golden colour.

To Serve:

Spread vegan butter over both sides of the buns and toast in a cast iron pan until crispy.

Serve immediately, piled with the cabbage, red onion, jalapeño, sambal mayo and pickles.

Nutrition:

Energy (calories): 918 kcal

Protein: 34.5 g

63%

Fat: 32.68 g

Carbohydrates: 126.19 g

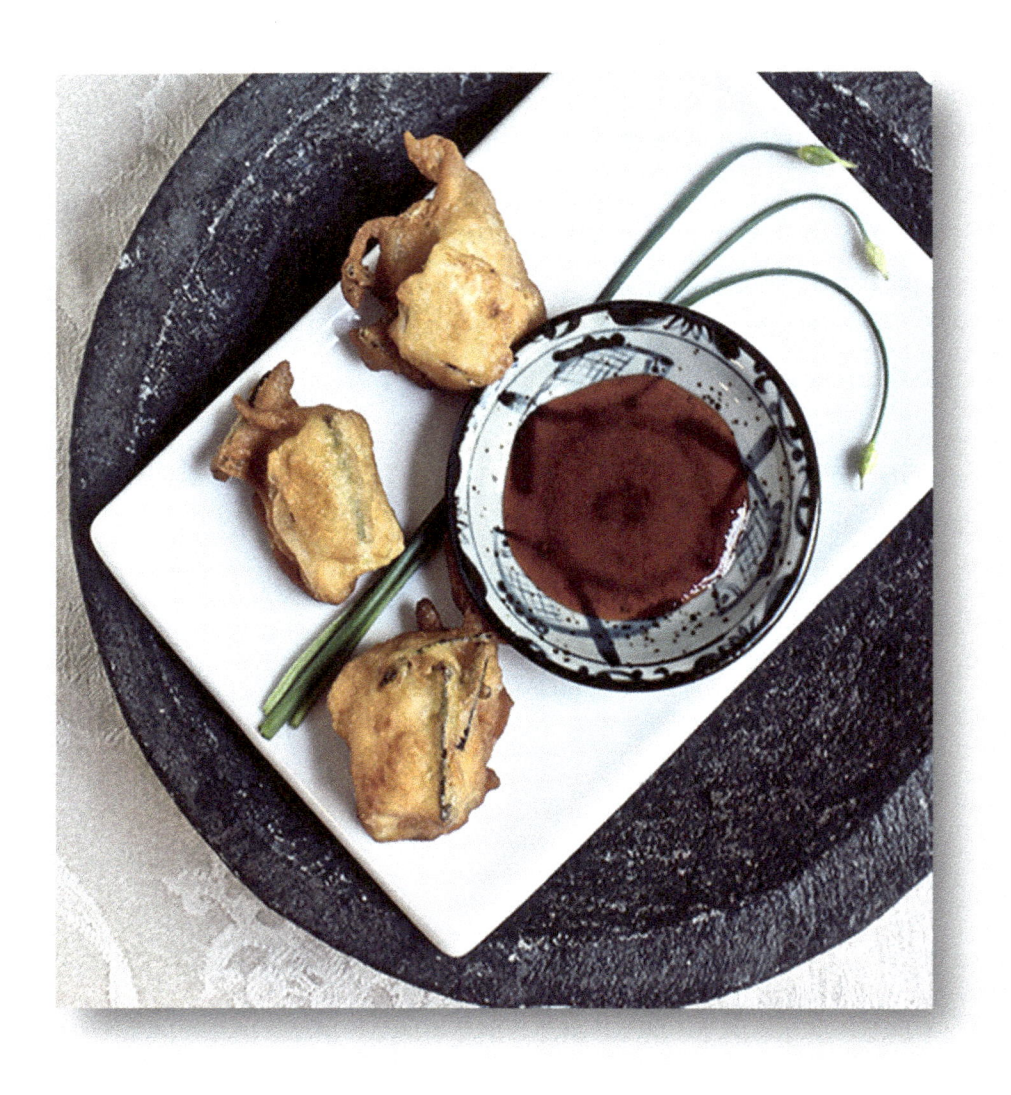

Lightning Source UK Ltd.
Milton Keynes UK
UKHW020807180621
385732UK00001B/104